AMERICAN WOMEN
images and realities

AMERICAN WOMEN

Images and Realities

Advisory Editors

ANNETTE K. BAXTER

LEON STEIN

A Note About This Volume

This study by Abraham Myerson, Professor of Neurology, Tufts College Medical School, sought to apply concepts of psychiatry in an effort to preserve mental health in the home while new freedoms and old restraints clashed there. A work of the early Twenties, it depicts the home as battle ground, the kitchen as stockade, housework as a heavy burden and the wife as incomplete woman. The book includes eleven studies of neurotic disorders in females.

THE NERVOUS HOUSEWIFE

BY

ABRAHAM MYERSON

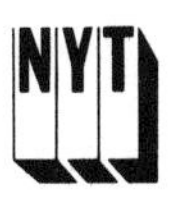

ARNO PRESS
A New York Times Company
New York • 1972

Reprint Edition 1972 by Arno Press Inc.

Copyright © 1920 by Little, Brown and Company
Reprinted by permission of Little, Brown and Company

Reprinted from a copy in The University of Illinois Library

American Women: Images and Realities
ISBN for complete set: 0-405-04445-3
See last pages of this volume for titles.

Manufactured in the United States of America

- - - - - - - - - - - - - -

Library of Congress Cataloging in Publication Data

Myerson, Abraham, 1881-1948.
The nervous housewife.

(American women: images and realities)
1. Woman--Health and hygiene. 2. Neurasthenia.
I. Title. II. Series.
RC351.M83 1972 616.8'528 72-2616
ISBN 0-405-04470-4

THE NERVOUS HOUSEWIFE

THE

NERVOUS HOUSEWIFE

BY

ABRAHAM MYERSON, M.D.

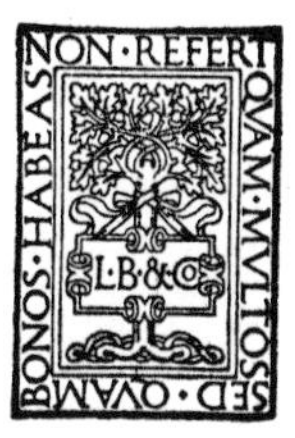

BOSTON

LITTLE, BROWN, AND COMPANY

1927

Copyright, 1920,

BY LITTLE, BROWN, AND COMPANY.

All rights reserved

PRINTED IN THE UNITED STATES OF AMERICA

CONTENTS

THE NERVOUS HOUSEWIFE

CHAPTER I

Introductory

How old is the problem of the Nervous Housewife?

Did the semi-mythical Cave Man (who is perhaps only a pseudo-scientific creation) on his return from a prehistoric hunt find his leafy spouse all in tears over her staglocythic house-cleaning, or the conduct of the youngest cave child? Did she complain of her back, did she have a headache every time they disagreed, did she fuss and fret until he lost his patience and dashed madly out to the Cave Man's Refuge?

We cannot tell; we only know that all humor aside, and without reference to the past, the Nervous Housewife is surely a phenomenon of the present-day American home. In greater or less degree she is in every man's home; nor is she alone the rich Housewife with too little to do, for though riches do not protect, poverty predisposes, and the poor Housewife is far more frequently the victim of this disease of occupation. Every practicing physician, every hospital clinic, finds her a problem, evoking pity, concern, exasperation, and despair. She goes from specialist to specialist, — orthopedic surgeon, gynecologist, X-ray man, neurologist. By the time she has completed a course of treatment she has tasted all the drugs in the pharmacopeia, wears plates on her feet, spectacles on her nose, has had her teeth tinkered with, and her insides straightened; has had a course in hydrotherapeutics, electrotherapeutics, osteopathy, and Christian Science!

Such is an extreme case; the minor cases pass through life burdened with pains and aches of the body and soul. And one of the commonest and saddest of transformations is the change of the gay, laughing young girl, radiant with love and all aglow at the thought of union with her man, into the housewife of a decade, — complaining, fatigued, and disillusioned. Bound to her husband by the ties the years and the children have brought, there is a wall of misunderstanding between them.

"Men don't understand," cries she. "Women are unreasonable," says he.

What are the causes of the change? Did the housewife of a past generation go through the same stage? Ask any man you meet and he will tell you his mother is or was more enduring than his wife. "She bore three times as many children; she did all her own housework; she baked more, cooked more, sewed more; she got up at five o'clock in the morning and went to bed at ten at night; she never went out, never had a vacation, did not know the meaning of manicure, pedicure, coiffure. She was contented, never extravagant, and rarely sick."

So the average man will say, and then: "Those were the good old days of simple living, gone like the dodo! To-day,—well, it reminds me of a joke I heard. One man meets another and says: 'By the way, I heard that your wife was the champion athlete at college.' 'Ah, yes,' said the husband; 'now she is too weak to wash the dishes.'

Is the average man's impression the correct one? Or are we dealing with the incorrigible disposition of man to glorify the past? To the majority of people their youth was an era of stronger, braver men, more wholesome, beautiful women. People were better, times were more natural, and there is a grim satisfaction in predicting that the "world is going to the dogs." "The good old days" has been the cry of man from the very earliest times.

Yet read what a contemporary of the housewife of three quarters of a century ago says, — the wisest, wittiest, sanest doctor of the day, Oliver Wendell Holmes. The genial autocrat of the breakfast table observes: "Talk about military duty! What is that to the warfare of a married maid of all work, with the title of mistress and an American female constitution which collapses just in the middle third of life, comes out vulcanized India rubber, if it happens to live through the period when health and strength are most wanted?"

And then, if one looks in the advertisements of half a century ago, one finds the nostrum dealer loudly proclaiming his capacity to cure what is evidently the Nervous Housewife. In America at least she has always existed, perhaps in lesser numbers than at present. And one remembers in a dim sort of way that the married woman of olden days was altogether faded at thirty-five, that she entered on middle life at a time when at least many of our women of to-day still think themselves young.

It becomes interesting and necessary at this point to trace the evolution of the home, because this is to trace the evolution of our housewife. We are apt to think of the home as originating in a sort of cave, where the little unit — the Man, the Woman, and the Children — dwelt in isolation, ever on the watch against marauders, either animal or human. In this cave the woman was the chattel of man; he had seized her by force and ruled by force.

Perhaps there was such a stage, but much more likely the home was a communal residence, where the man-herd, the group, the clan, the Family in the larger sense dwelt. Only a large group would be safe, and the strong social instinct, the herd feeling, was the basis of the home. Here the men and women dwelt in a promiscuity that through the ages went through an evolution which finally became the father-controlled monogamy of to-day. Here the women lived; here they span, sewed, built; here they started the arts, the handicrafts, and the religions. And from here the men went forth to fish and hunt and fight, grim males to whom a maiden was a thing to court and a wife a thing to enslave.

Just how the home became more and more segregated and the family life more individualized is not in the province of this book to detail. This is certain: that the home was not only a place where man and woman mated, where their children were born and reared, where food was prepared and cooked, and where shelter from the elements was obtained; it was also the first great workshop, where all the manifold industries had their inception and early development. The housewife was then not only mother, wife, cook, and nurse; she was the spinner, the weaver, the tanner, the dyer, the brewer, the druggist.

Even in the high civilization of the Jews this wide scope of the housewife prevailed.

Read what the wisest, perhaps because most married, of men says:

She seeketh wool and flax,
And worketh willingly with her hands.
She is like the merchant ships;
She bringeth her food from afar.
She considereth a field, and buyeth it.
With the fruit of her hands she planteth a vineyard.
She girdeth her loins with strength,
And maketh strong her arms.
She perceiveth that her merchandise is good.
Her lamp goeth not out by night.
She layeth her hands to the distaff
And her hands hold the spindle.

. . . .

She is not afraid of the snow for her household:
For all her household are clothed with scarlet.
She maketh for herself coverlets,
She maketh linen garments and selleth them,
And delivereth girdles unto the merchants.

No wonder "her children rise up and call her blessed" and it is somewhat condescending of her husband when he "praiseth her." All we learn of him is that he "is known in the gates when he sitteth among the elders of the land." With a wife like her, this was all he had to do.

This combination of industrialism and

domesticity continued until gradually men stepped into the field of work, perhaps as a result of their wives' example, and became farmers on a larger scale, merchants of a wider scope, artisans, handicraftsmen, guild members of a more developed technique. Woman started these things in the home or near it; man, through his restless energy, specialized and thus developed an intenser civilization. But even up till the nineteenth century woman carried on all her occupations at the home, which still continued to be workshop and hearth.

Then man invented the machine, harnessed steam, wired electricity, and there was born the Factory, the specialized house of industry, in which there works no artisan, only factory hands. The home could not compete with this man's monster, into which flowed one river of raw material and out of which poured another of finished products. But not only did the factory dye, weave, spin, tan, etc.; it also invaded the innermost sphere of woman's work. For her loaf of bread it turned out thousands, until finally she is beginning to give up baking; for her hit-or-miss jellies, preserves, jams, it invented scientific canning with absolute methods, handy forms, tempting flavors. And canning did not stop there; meats, soups, vegetables, fruits are now placed in the hands of the housewife "Ready to Serve," until the cynical now state, "Woman is no longer a cook, she is a can opener." With all the talk in this modern time of women invading man's field, it is just to remark that man has stepped into woman's work and carried off a huge part of it to his own creation, the factory.

Thus it has come to pass that in our day the housewife does but little dyeing, spinning, weaving, is no longer a handicraftsman, and in addition is turning over a large part of her food preparation and cooking to the factory.

But the factory is not content with thus disarranging the ancient scheme of things by invading the housewife's province; it has dragged a large number of women, yearly increasing in number and proportion, into industry. Thus it has made this condition of affairs: that it takes the young girl from the home for the few years that intervene before her marriage. She is thus initiated into wage-earning before she becomes a man's wife, the housewife.

This industrial period of a girl's life is important psychologically, for it profoundly influences her reaction to her status and work as homekeeper.

Of even greater importance to our study than the influence of the factory is the rise of what is known as feminism. Of all the living creatures in the world the female of the human species has been the most downtrodden, for to every wretched class of man there was a still inferior, more wretched group, their wives. She was a slave to the slaves, a dependent of the abjectly poor. When men passed through the stage where woman's life might be taken at a whim, she remained a creature without rights of the wider kind. Men debated whether she had a soul, made cynical proverbs about her, called her the "weaker vessel," and debarred her from political and economic equality, classing her up to this very moment in rights with the idiot, the imbecile, and the criminal. Worse than this, they gave her a spurious homage, created a lop-sided chivalry, and caused her to accept as her ideal goal of womanhood the achievement of beauty and the entrance into wifehood. After they tied her hand and foot with restrictions and belittling ideals, they capped the climax by calling her weak and petty by nature and even got her to believe it!

It is not my intention to trace the rise of feminism. Brave women arose from age to age to glorify the world and their sex, and men here and there championed them. Man started to emancipate himself from slavery, and noble ideals of the equality of mankind first were whispered, then shouted as battle cries, and finally chiseled with enduring letters into the foundations of States. "But if all this was good for men, why not for women — why should they be fettered by illiteracy, pettiness, dependence; why should they be voiceless in the state and world?" So asked the feminists. The factory called for women as labor; they became the clerks, the teachers, the typists, the nurses. Medicine and the law opened their doors, at least in part. And now we are on the verge of universal suffrage, with women entering into the affairs of the world, theoretically at least the equals of man.

But with the entrance of woman into many varied professions and occupations, with a wider access to experience and knowledge, arose what may be called the era of the "individualization of woman." For if any group of people are kept under more or less uniform conditions in early life, if one goal is held out as the only legitimate aim and end, in a word, if their training and purposes are made alike, they become alike and individuality never develops. With individuality comes rebellion at old-established conditions, dissatisfaction, discontent, and especially if the old ideal still remains in force. This new type of woman is not so well fitted for the old type of marriage as her predecessors. There arises a group of consequences based psychologically on this, a fact which we shall find of great importance later on.

Women still regard marriage as their chief goal in life, still enter homes, still bear children, and take their husband's name. But having become more individualized they demand more definite individual treatment and rebel more at what they consider an infringement of their rights as human beings. Also, and unfortunately, they still wish the right to be whimsical, they continue to reserve for themselves the weapons of tears, reproaches, and unreasonable demands. This has brought about the divorce evil.

Briefly the "divorce" evil arises first from the rebellion of woman against marital drunkenness, unfaithfulness, neglect, brutality that a former generation of wives tolerated and even expected. Second, it arises from a conflict between the institution of marriage which still carries with it the chattel idea — that woman is property — and a generation of women that does not accept this. Third, it arises from the ill-balanced demands of women to be treated as equals and also as irresponsible, petty, and indulged tyrants. Men are unable to adjust themselves to the shattering of the romantic ideal, and the home disintegrates. Though divorce is the top of the crest of marital unhappiness, it really represents only the extreme cases, and behind it is a huge body of quarreling and divided homes.

We shall later see that our Nervous Housewife has symptoms and pains and aches and changes in mood and feeling that are born of the conflict that is in part pictured by divorce. *Divorce is a manifestation of the discontent of women, and so is the nervousness of the housewife.*

There arises as a result of this individualization of woman, as a result of increasing physiological knowledge, the hugely important fact of restricted child bearing. The woman will no longer bear children indiscriminately, — and the large family is soon to be a thing of the past in America and in all the civilized world. The-woman-that-knows-how shrinks from the long nine months of pregnancy, the agony of the birth, and the weary restricted months of nursing. Had the woman of a past time known how, she too would have refused to bear. In this the housewife of to-day is seconded by her husband, for where he has sympathy for his wife he prefers to let her decide the number of children, and also he is impressed by the high cost of rearing them.

One gets cynical about the influence of church, patriotism, and press when one sees how the housewife has disregarded these influences. For all the religions preach that race suicide is a sin, all the statesmen point out that only decadent nations restrict families, and all or nearly all the press thunder against it. It is even against the law for a physician or other person to instruct in the methods of birth restriction, and yet — the birth rate steadily drops. An immigrant mother has six, eight, or ten children and her daughter has one, two, or three, very rarely more, and often enough none. This is true even of races close to religious teaching, such as the Irish Catholic and the Jew.

One can well be cynical of the power of religion and teaching and law when one finds that even the families of ministers, rabbis, editors, and lawmakers, all of whom stand publicly for natural birth, have shown a great reduction in their size, that has taken place in a single generation.

Is the modern woman more susceptible to the effects of pregnancy, — less resistant to the strain of childbearing and childbirth? It is a quite general impression amongst obstetricians that this is a fact and also that fewer women are able to nurse their babies. If so, these phenomena are of the highest importance to the race and likewise to the problem of the new housewife. For we shall learn that the lowering of energy is both a cause and symptom of her neuroses.

If then we summarize what has been thus far outlined, we find two currents in the evolution of the housewife. *First,* she has yielded a large part of her work to the factory, practically all of that part of it which is industrial and a considerable portion of the food preparation.

Second, there has been a rise in the dignity and position of woman in the past one hundred and fifty years which has had many results. She has considerably widened the scope of her experience with life through work in the factory, in the office, in the schoolhouse, and in the professions. This has changed her attitude toward her original occupation of housewife and is a psychological fact of great importance. She has become more industrial and individualized, and as a result has declined to live in unsatisfactory relations with man, so that divorce has become more frequent. In part this is also caused by her inability to give up petty irresponsibility while claiming equality. Finally, the declining birth rate is still further evidence of her individualization and is in a sense her denial of mere femaleness and an affirmation of freedom.

CHAPTER II

The Nature of "Nervousness"

Preliminary to our discussion of the nervousness of the housewife we must take up without great regard to details the subject of nervousness in general.

Nervousness, like many another word of common speech, has no place whatever in medicine. Indeed, no term indicating an abnormal condition is so loosely used as this one.

People say a man is nervous when they mean he is subject to attacks of anger, an emotional state. Likewise he is nervous when he is a victim of fear, a state literally the opposite of the first. Or, if he is restless, is given to little tricks like pulling at his hair, or biting his nails, he is nervous. The mother excuses her spoiled child on the ground of his nervousness, and I have seen a thoroughly bad boy who branded his baby sister with a heated spoon called "nervous." A "nervous breakdown" is a familiar verbal disguise for one or other of the sinister faces of insanity itself.

It should be made clear that what we are dealing with in the nervous housewife is not a special form of nervous disorder. It conforms to the general types found in single women and also in men. It differs in the intensity of symptoms, in the way they group themselves, and in the causes.

Physicians use the term psychoneuroses to include a group of nervous disorders of so-called functional nature. That is to say, there is no alteration that can be found in the brain, the spinal cord, or any part of the nervous system. In this, these conditions differ from such diseases as locomotor ataxia, tumor of the brain, cerebral hemorrhage, etc., because there are marked changes in the structure in the latter troubles. One might compare the psychoneuroses to a watch which needed oiling or cleaning, or merely a winding up, — as against one in which a vital part was broken.

The most important of the psychoneuroses, in so far as the housewife is concerned, is the condition called neurasthenia, although two other diseases, psychasthenia and hysteria, are of importance.

It is interesting that neurasthenia is considered by many physicians as a disease of modern times. Indeed, it was first described in 1869 by the eminent neurologist Beard, who thought it was entirely caused by the stress and strain of American life. That not only America, but every part of the whole civilized world has its neurasthenia is now an accepted fact. Knowing what we do of its causes we infer that it is probably as old as mankind; but there exists no reasonable doubt that modern life, with its hurry, its tensions, its widespread and ever present excitement, has increased the proportion of people involved.

Particularly the increase in the size and number of the cities, as compared with the country, is a great factor in the spread of neurasthenia. Then, too, the introduction of so-called time-saving, *i.e.* distance-annihilating instruments, such as the telephone, telegraph, railroad, etc., have acted not so much to save time as to increase the number of things done, seen, and heard. The busy man with his telephone close at hand may be saving time on each transaction, but by enormously increasing the number of his transactions he is not saving *himself.*

The keynote of neurasthenia is *increased liability to fatigue.* The tired feeling that comes on with a minimum of exertion, worse on arising than on going to bed, is its distinguishing mark. Sleep, which should remove the fatigue of the day, does not; the victim takes half of his day to get going; and at night, when he should have the delicious drowsiness of bedtime, he is wide-awake and disinclined to go to bed or sleep. This fatigue enters into all functions of the mind and body. Fatigue of mind brings about lack of concentration, an inattention; and this brings about an inefficiency that worries the patient beyond words as portending a mental breakdown. Fatigue of purpose brings a listlessness of effort, a shirking of the strenuous, the more distressing because the victim is often enough an idealist with over-lofty purposes. Fatigue of mood is marked by depression of a mild kind, a liability to worry, an unenthusiasm for those one loves or for the things formerly held dearest. And finally the fatigue is often marked by a lack of control over the emotional expression, so that anger blazes forth more easily over trifles, and the tears come upon even a slight vexation. *To be neurasthenic is to magnify the pins and pricks of life into calamities, and to be the victim of an abnormal state that is neither health nor disease.*

The more purely physical symptoms constitute almost everything imaginable.

1. Pains and aches of all kinds stand out prominently; headache, backache, pains in the shoulders and arms, pains in the feet and legs, pains that flit here and there, dull weary pains, disagreeable feelings rather than true pains. These pains are frequently related to disagreeable experiences and thoughts, but it is probable that fatigue plays the principal part in evoking them.

2. Changes in the appetite, in the condition of the stomach and bowels, are prominent. Loss of appetite is complained of, or more often a capricious appetite, vanishing quickly, or else too easily satisfied. The capriciousness of appetite is undoubtedly emotional, for disagreeable emotions, such as worry,

fear, vexation, have long been known as the chief enemies of appetite.

With this change of appetite goes a host of disorders manifested by "belching", "sour stomach", "logy feelings", etc. What is back of these lay terms is that the tone, movement, and secreting activity of the stomach is impaired in neurasthenia. When we consider later on the nature of emotion, we shall find these changes to be part of the disorder of emotion.

3. So, too, there is constipation. In how far the constipation is primary and in how far it is secondary is a question. At any rate, once it is established, it interferes with all the functions of the organism by its interference with the mood.

The following story of Voltaire bluntly illustrates a fact of widespread knowledge. Voltaire and an Englishman, after an intimate philosophical discussion, decided that the aches and pains of life outnumbered the agreeable sensations, and that to live was to endure unhappiness. Therefore, they decided that jointly they would commit suicide and named the time and the place. On the day appointed the Englishman appeared with a revolver ready to blow out his brains, but no Voltaire was to be seen. He looked high and low and then went to the sage's home. There he found him seated before a table groaning with the good things of life and reading a naughty novel with an expression of utmost enjoyment. Said the Englishman to Voltaire, "This was the day upon which we were to commit suicide." "Ah, yes," said Voltaire, "so we were, but to-day my bowels moved well."

4. The disturbed sleep, either as insomnia or an unrestful, dream-disturbed slumber, is a distressing symptom. For we look to the bed as a refuge from our troubles, as a sanctuary wherein is rebuilded our strength. We may link work and sleep as the two complementary functions necessary for happiness. If sleep is disturbed, so is work, and with that our purposes are threatened. So disturbed sleep has not only its bodily effects but has its marked results on our happiness.

5. Fundamental in the symptoms of neurasthenia is fear. This fear takes two main forms. First, the worry over the life situation in general, that is to say, fear concerning business; fear concerning the health

and prosperity of the household; fear that magnifies anything that has even the faintest possibility of being direful into something that is almost sure to happen and be disastrous. This constant worry over the possibilities of the future is both a cause of neurasthenia and a symptom, in that once a neurasthenic state is established, the liability to worry becomes greatly increased.

Second, there is a special form of worry called by the old authors hypochondriacism, which essentially is fear about one's own health. The hypochondriac magnifies every flutter of his heart into heart disease, every stitch in his side into pleurisy, every cough into tuberculosis, every pain in the abdomen into cancer of the stomach, every headache into the possibility of brain tumor or insanity. He turns his gaze inward upon himself, and by so doing becomes aware of a host of sensations that otherwise stream along unnoticed. Our vision was meant for the environment, for the world in which we live, since the bodily processes go on best unnoticed. The little fugitive pains and aches; the little changes in respiration; the rumblings and movements of the gastro-intestinal tract have no essential meaning in the majority of cases, but once they are watched with apprehension and anxiety, they multiply extraordinarily in number and intensity. One of the cardinal groups of symptoms in a neurasthenic is this fear of serious bodily disease for which he seeks examination and advice constantly. Naturally enough, he becomes the choicest prey for the charlatan, the faker, or perhaps ranks second to the victim of venereal or sexual disease. The faker usually assures him that he has the disorders he fears and then proceeds to cure him by his own expensive and marvelous course of treatment.

What has been sketched here is merely the outside of neurasthenia. Back of it as causative are matters we shall deal with in detail later on in relation to the housewife,— matters like innate temperament, bad training, liability to worry, wounded pride, failure, desire for sympathy, monotony of life, boredom, unhappiness, pessimism of outlook, over-æsthetic tastes, unfulfilled and thwarted desires, secret jealousy, passions and longings, fear of death, sex problems and difficulties and doubt; matters like recent illness, childbirth, poverty, overwork, wrong sex habits, lack of fresh air, etc.

Fundamentally neurasthenia is a deënergization. By this is meant that either there is an actual reduction in the energy of the body (as after a sickness, pregnancy, etc.) or else something impedes the discharge of energy. This latter is usually an emotional matter, or arises from some thought, some life situation of a depressing kind.

It is necessary and important that we consider these two aspects of our subject a little closer, not so much as regards the housewife, but over the wider field of the human being.

The human being, like every living thing, is an instrument for the building up and discharge of energy. He takes in food, the food is digested (made over into certain substances) and these are built up into the tissues, — and then their energy is discharged as heat and as motion. The heat is the body temperature, the motion is the movement of the human body in all the marvelous variety of which it is capable. In other words, the discharge of energy is the play of our childhood and of our later years; it is the skill and strength of our arms, the cleverness of our hands, the fleetness of our feet, the joyous vigor of our love-making, the embrace; it is the noble purpose, the long, hard-fought battles of any kind. It is all that is summed up in desire, purpose, and achievement.

Now all these things may be impeded by actual reduction of energy, as in tuberculosis, cancer, or in the lassitude of convalescence. In addition there are emotions, feelings, thoughts that energize, — that create vigor and strength of body and mind. Joy rouses the spirit; one dances, laughs, sings, shouts; or the more quiet type of person takes up work with zeal and renewed energy. Hope brings with it an eagerness for the battle, a zest for work. The glow of pride that comes with praise is a stimulus of great power and enlarges the scope of the personality. The feeling that comes with successful effort, with rewarded effort, is a new birth of purpose and will. And whatever arouses the fighting spirit, which in the last analysis is based on anger, achieves the same end.

There are *deënergizing emotions and experiences* as well, things that suddenly rob the victim of strength and purpose. Fear of a certain type is one of these things, as when one's knees knock together, the limbs become as it were without the control of the will, the heart flutters, and the voice is hoarse and weak. Fear of sickness, fear of death, either for one's self or some beloved one, may completely deënergize the strongest man. Then there is hope deferred, and disappointment, the frustration of desire and purpose, helplessness before insult and injustice, blame merited or unmerited, the feeling of failure and inevitable disaster. There is the unhappy life situation, — the mistaken marriage, the disillusionment of betrayed love, the dashing of parental pride. The profoundest deënergization of life may come from a failure of interest in one's work, a boredom due to monotony, a dropping out of enthusiasm from the mere failure of new stimuli, as occurs with loneliness. Any or all of these factors may bring about a neurasthenic, deenergized state with lowering of the functions of mind and body. We shall discover how this comes about farther on.

What part does a subconscious personality take in all this and in further symptoms? Is there a subconsciousness, and what is it?

In answer, the majority of modern psychologists and psychopathologists affirm the existence of a subconscious personality. One needs only mention James, Janet, Ribot, McDougall, Freud, Prince, out of a host of writers. Whether they are right or not, or whether we now deal with a new fashion in mental science, this can be affirmed — that every human being is a pot boiling with desires, passions, lusts, wishes, purposes, ideas, and emotions, some of which he clearly recognizes and clearly admits, and some of which he does not clearly recognize and which he would deny.

These desires, passions, purposes, etc., are not in harmony one with another; they are often irreconcilable and one has to be smothered for the sake of the other. Thus a sex feeling that is not legitimate, an illicit forbidden love has to be conquered for the sake of the purpose to be religious or good, or the desire to be respected. So one may struggle against a hatred for a person whom one should love, — a husband, a wife, an invalid parent, or child whose care is a burden, and one refuses to recognize that there is such a struggle. So one may seek to suppress jealousy, envy of the nearest and dearest; soul-stirring, forbidden passions; secret revolt against morality and law which may (and often do) rage in the most puritanical breast.

In the theory of the subconscious these undesired thoughts, feelings, passions, wishes, are repressed and pushed into the innermost recesses of the being, out of the light of the conscious personality, but nevertheless acting on the personality, distorting it, wearying it.

However this may be, there is struggle, conflict in every human breast and especially difficult and undecided struggles in the case of the neurasthenic. Literally, secretly or otherwise, he is a house divided against himself, deënergized by fear, disgust, revolt, and conflict.

And the housewife we are trying to understand is particularly such a creature, with a host of deënergizing influences playing on her, buffeting her. Our aim will be to analyze these influences and to discover how they work.

I have stated that in medical practice two other types are described, — psychasthenia and hysteria. These are not so definitely related to the happenings of life as to the inborn disposition of the patient. Nor are they quite so common in the housewife as the neurasthenic, deënergized state. However, they are usually of more serious nature, and as such merit a description.

By the term psychasthenia is understood a group of conditions in which the bodily symptoms, such as fatigue, sleeplessness, loss of appetite, etc., are either not so marked as in neurasthenia, or else are overshadowed by other, more distinctly mental symptoms.

These mental symptoms are of three main types. There is a tendency to recurring fears, — fears of open places, fears of closed places, fear of leaving home, of being alone, fear of eating or sleeping, fear of dirt, so that the victim is impelled continually to wash the hands, fear of disease — especially such as syphilis — and a host of other fears, all of which are recognized as unreasonable, against which the victim struggles but vainly. Sometimes the fear is nameless, vague, undifferentiated, and comes on like a cloud with rapid heartbeat, faint feelings, and a sense of impending death. Sometimes the fear is related to something that has actually happened, as, fear of anything hot after a sunstroke; or fear of any vehicle after an automobile accident.

There is also a tendency to obsessive ideas and doubts; that is, ideas and doubts that persist in coming against the will of the patient, such as the obscene word or phrase that continually obtrudes itself on a chaste woman, or the doubt whether one has shut the door or properly turned off the gas. Of course, everybody has such obsessions and doubts occasionally, but to be psychasthenic about it is to have them continually and to have them obtrude themselves into every action. In extreme psychasthenia the difficulty of "making up the mind", of deciding, becomes so great that a person may suffer agonies of internal debate about crossing the street, putting on his clothes, eating his meals, doing his work, about every detail of his coming, going, doing, and thinking. A restless anxiety results, a fear of insanity, an inefficiency, and an incapacity for sustained effort that results in the name that is often applied, — "anxiety neurosis."

Third, there is a group of impulsions and habits. Citing a few absurd impulsions: a person feels compelled to step over every crack, to touch the posts along his journey, to take the stairs three steps at a time. The habits range from the queer desire to bite one's nails to the quick that is so common in children and which persists in the psychasthenic adult, to the odd grimaces and facial contortions, blinking eyes and cracking joints of the inveterate *ticquer*. Against some of these habit spasms, comparable to severe stammering, all measures are in vain, for there seems to be a queer pleasure in these acts against which the will of the patient is powerless.

Especially do the first two described types of trouble follow exhaustion, acute illness, sudden fright, and long painful ordeal. The ground is prepared for these conditions, *e.g.* by the strain of long attendance on a sick husband or child. Then, suddenly one day, comes a queer fear or a faint dizzy feeling which awakens great alarm, is brooded upon, wondered at, and its return feared. This fearful expectation really makes the return inevitable, and then the disease starts. If the patient would seek competent advice at this stage, recovery would usually be prompt. Instead, there is a long unsuccessful struggle, with each defeat tending to make the fear or anxiety or obsession habitual. Sometimes, perhaps in most cases, and in all cases according to Freud and his followers, there is a long-hidden series of causes behind the symptoms; subconscious sexual conflicts and repressions, etc. It may be stated here that the present author is not at all a Freudian and believes that the causes of these forms of nervousness are simpler, more related to the big obvious factors in life, than to the curiously complicated and bizarrely sexual Freudian factors. People get tired, disgusted, apprehensive; they hate where they should love; love where they should hate; are jealous unreasonably; are bored, tortured by monotony; have their hopes, purposes, and desires frustrated and blocked; fear death and old age, however brave a face they may wear; want happiness and achievement, and some break, one way or another, according to their emotional and intellectual resistance. These and other causes are the great factors of the conditions we have been considering.

Of all the forms of nervousness proper, the psychoneuroses, hysteria is probably the one having its source mainly in the character of the patient. That is to say, outward happenings play a part which is secondary to the personality defect. Hysteria is one of the oldest of diseases and has probably played a very important rôle in the history of man. Unquestionably many of the religions have depended upon hysteria, for it is in this field that "miracle cures" occur. All founders of religions have based part of their claim on the belief of others in their healing power. Nothing is so spectacular as when the hysterical blind see, the hysterical dumb talk, the hysterical cripple throws away his crutches and walks. In every age and in every country, in every faith, there have been the equivalents of Lourdes and St. Anne de Beaupré.

In hysteria four important groups of symptoms occur in the housewife as well as in her single sisters and brothers.

There is first of all an emotional instability, with a tendency to prolonged and freakish manifestations, — the well-known hysterics with laughing, crying, etc. Fundamental in the personality of the hysterics is this instability, this emotionality, which is however secondary to an egotistic, easily wounded nature, craving sympathy and respect and often unable legitimately to earn them.

A group of symptoms that seem hard to explain are the so-called paralyses. These paralyses may affect almost any part, may come in a moment and go as suddenly, or last for years. They may concern arm, leg, face, hands, feet, speech, etc. They seem very severe, but are due to worry, to misdirected ideas and emotions and not at all to injury to the nervous system. They are manifestations of what the neurologists call "dissociations of the personality." That is, conflicts of emotions, ideas, and purposes of the type previously described have occurred, and a paralysis has resulted. These paralyses yield remarkably to any energizing influence like good fortune, the compelling personality of a physician or clergyman or healer (the miracle cure), or a serious danger. The latter is exemplified in the cases now and then reported of people who have not been out of bed for years, but are aroused by threat of some danger, like a fire, reach safety, and thereafter are well.

Similar in type to the paralyses are losses

of sensation in various parts of the body, — losses so complete that one may thrust a needle deep into the flesh without pain to the patient. In the days of witch-hunting the witch-hunters would test the women suspected with a pin, and if they found places where pain was not felt, considered they had proof of witchcraft or diabolic possession, so that many a hysteric was hanged or drowned. The history of man is full of psychopathic characters and happenings; insane men have changed the course of human events by their ideas and delusions, and on the other hand society has continually mistaken the insane and the nervously afflicted for criminals or wretches deserving severest punishment.

Especially striking in hysteria are the curious changes in consciousness that take place. These range from what seem to be fainting spells to long trances lasting perhaps for months, in which animation is apparently suspended and the body seems on the brink of death. In olden days the Delphian oracles were people who had the power voluntarily of throwing themselves into these hysteric states and their vague statements were taken to be heaven-inspired. To-day, their descendants in hysteria are the crystal gazers, the mediums, the automatic writers that by a mixture of hysteria and faking deceive the simple and credulous.

For, in the last analysis, all hysterics are deceivers both of themselves and of others. Their symptoms, real enough at bottom, are theatrical and designed for effect. As I shall later show, they are weapons, used to gain an end, which is the whim or will of the patient.

In order to clinch our understanding of the above conditions we must now consider in more detail certain phases of emotion.

Fear curdles the blood, anger floods the body with passion, sorrow flexes the proud head to earth and stifles the heartbeat; joy opens the floodgates of strength, and hope lifts up the head and braces man's soul.

Man is said to be a rational being, but his thought is directed mainly against the problems of nature, much more rarely against *his own* problems. It is for emotion that we live, for emotion in the wide sense of pleasure and pride. What guides us in our conduct is desire, and desire in the last analysis is based on the instincts and the allied emotions, — hunger, sex, property, competition, co-operation. The intelligence guides the instincts and governs the emotions, but in the case of the vast majority of mankind is swept out of the field when any great decision is to be made.

We are accustomed to thinking of emotion as a thing purely psychical, — purely of the mind, despite the fact that all the great descriptions and all the homely sayings portray it as bodily. "My heart thumped like a steam engine," or "I could not catch my breath"; "a cold chill played up and down my back"; "I swallowed hard, because my mouth was so dry I could not speak." And the Bible repeatedly says of the man stricken by fear, "His bowels turned to water," with a graphic force only equaled by its truth.

William James, nearly simultaneously with Lange, pointed out that emotion cannot be separated from its physical concomitants and maintain its identity. That is, if we separate in our minds the weak, chilly feeling, the dry mouth, the racing heart, the sharp, harsh breathing, and the tension of the muscles getting ready for flight from the feeling of fear, nothing tangible is left. Similarly with sorrow or joy or anger. Take the latter emotion; imagine yourself angry, — immediately the jaw becomes set and the lips draw back in a semi-snarl, the fists clench and the muscles tighten, while the head and body are thrust forward in what is, as Darwin pointed out, the preparation for pouncing on the foe. Even if you mimic anger without any especial reason, there steals over you a feeling not unlike anger.

In a famous paragraph James essentially states that instead of crying because we are sorry, it is fully as likely that we are sorry because we cry. So with every emotion; we are afraid because we run away, and happy because we dance and shout. In other words he reversed the order of things as the every-day person would see it; makes primary and of fundamental importance the physical response rather than the feeling itself.

This has been widely disagreed with, and is not at all an acceptable theory in its entirety. Yet modern physiology has shown that emotion is largely a physical matter, largely a thing of blood vessels, heartbeat, lungs, glands, and digestive organs. This physical foundation of emotion is a very important matter in our study of the housewife as of every other living person. For it is especially in the emotional disturbance that the origin of much of nervousness is to be found, and that on what may be called the physical basis of emotion.

What can emotion produce that is pathological, detrimental to well-being? We may start with the grossest, simplest manifestations. It may entirely upset digestion, as in the vomiting of disgust and excitement. Or, in lesser measure, it may completely destroy the appetite, as occurs when a disturbing emotion arises at mealtime. This is probably brought about by the checking of the gastric secretions. (Cannon's work; Pavlow's work.)

It may check the secretion of milk in the nursing mother, or it may change the quality of the milk so that it almost poisons the infant. It may cause the bladder and bowels to be evacuated, or it may prevent their evacuation.

It may so change the supply of blood in the body as to leave the head without sufficient quantity and thus bring about a fainting spell; *i.e.* may absolutely deprive the victim of consciousness. In lesser degree it causes the blush, a visible manifestation of emotion often very distressing.

It may completely abolish sex power in the male, or it may bring about sex manifestations which the victim would almost rather die than show.

It may completely deënergize so that neither interest, enthusiasm, or power remains. This is a familiar effect of sorrow but occurs in lesser degree with the form of fear called worry.

The fact is that emotion is an intense bodily response to a situation which when perceived is the state of feeling. This intense bodily response, involving the very minutest tissues of the body, may increase the available energy, may help the bodily functioning, may stimulate the "psychical" processes, but also it may deënergize to an extraordinary degree, it may interfere with every function, including thought and action. It may surely produce acute illness, and it may, though rarely, produce death.

Moreover, it is extraordinarily contagious. Every one knows how a hearty laugh spreads, and how quick the response to a smile. Indeed, emotion has probably for one of its main functions the producing of an effect on some one else, and all the world uses emotion for this purpose. Anger is used to produce fear, sorrow to evoke sympathy, fear is to bring about relenting, a smile and laughter, friendliness, except where one smiles or laughs *at* some one, and then its design is to bring sorrow, anger, or pain. The leader maintains a hopeful, joyous demeanor so that his followers may also be joyous or hopeful and thus be energized to their best. Morale is the state of emotion of a group; it is raised when joyous, energizing emotions are set working in the group and is lowered when pessimistic deënergizing emotions become dominant. A city or a nation becomes energized with good news and success and de-energized when the battle seems lost.

The spread of emotion from person to person by sympathetic feeling or the reverse (as when we get depressed because our enemy is happy) is a social fact of incalculable importance. The problem of the nervous housewife is a problem of society because she gives her mood over to her family or else intensely dissatisfies its members so that the home ties are greatly weakened.

This spread of emotion was happily portrayed by a motion picture I recently saw. Old Grouchy Moneybags, wealthy beyond measure and afflicted with gout, is seated at his breakfast table. In the next room, seen with the all-seeing eye of the movie, the butler makes love to the very willing maid. In the kitchen the fat cook is feeding the ever hungry butcher's boy with gingerbread and cake, and on the back steps the household cat is purring gently in contentment. Happiness is the predominant note.

Then Old Moneybags savagely rings the bell. Enters the butler, obsequious and solicitous. "The coffee is bad, the toast is vile, everything is wrong. You are a *deleted deleted deleted deleted* rascal." Exit the butler, outwardly humble, inwardly a raging flood of anger, and he meets the maid, who archly invites his attentions. She gets them, only they are in the form of an angry shove and an oath. White with indignation, she stamps her foot and runs into the kitchen, bursting into tears. The cook, solicitous, receives a slap in the face, and as the maid bounces out, the cook, seeking a victim, grabs away the gingerbread from the butcher's boy.

And that still hungry juvenile slams the door as he leaves and kicks the slumbering cat off the back doorstep.

Unfortunately the film did not show what the outraged cat did. Possibly it started a devastation that reached back into Money-bags' career; at any rate the unusual little picture (which later went on to the usual happy ending) showed how emotion spreads through the world, just as disease does. The infection that starts in the hovel finally strikes down the rich man's child, enthroned in the palace. The mood engendered by the humiliation of poverty or cruelty or any injustice finally shakes a king off his throne.

So when we trace the deënergizing emotions of the housewife, we are tracing factors that affect her husband, his work, and Society at large; we trace the things that mold her children, and thus we follow her mood, her emotion, into the future, into history.

CHAPTER III

Types of Housewife Predisposed to Nervousness

There are three main factors in the production of the nervousness of the housewife, and they weave and interweave in a very complex way to produce a variety of results. All the things of life, no matter how simple in appearance, are a complex combination of action and reaction. Our housewife's symptoms are no exception, whether they are mainly pains, aches, and fatigue, or the deeply motivated doubt or feeling of unreality.

The nature of the housewife, the conditions of her life, and her relations to her husband are these three factors. All enter into each case, though in some only one may be emphasized as of importance. There are cases where the nature of the woman is mainly the essential cause, others where it is the conditions of her life, and still others where the husband stands out as the source of her symptoms.

We are now to consider the nature of the housewife as our first factor. We may preamble this by saying that a woman essentially normal in one relationship in life may be abnormal in some other, may be the traditional square peg in the round hole. Moreover, we are to insist on the essential and increasing individuality of women, which is to a large extent a recent phenomenon. The cynical commonplace is "All women are alike" — and then follows the specific accusation — "in fickleness", "in extravagance", "in unreasonableness", in this trick or that. The chief effort of conservatism is to make them alike, to fit each one for the same life by the same training in habits, knowledge, abilities, and ideals.

Talk about Prussianism! The great Prussianism, with its ideal of uniformity, serviceability, and servility, has been the masculine ideal of woman's life. Man was to be diversified as life itself, was to taste all its experiences, but woman had her sphere, which belied all mathematics by being a narrow groove.

The nineteenth century changed all that, — or started the change which is going on with extraordinary rapidity in the twentieth. There are all kinds of women, at least potentially. It may be true that woman tends less to vary than man, that she follows a conservative middle-of-the-road biologically, while man spreads out, but no one can be sure of this until woman's early training to some extent resembles man's.

1. From the very start woman is trained to vanity. Every mother loves to doll up her girl baby, and the child is admired for her dress and appearance. Now it is an essential quality of the normal human being that he accepts as an ideal the quality most admired. To the young child, the girl, the young woman, the important thing is Looks, Looks, Looks! The first question asked about a woman is, "Is she pretty?" The pretty girls, the ones most courted, the ones surest on the whole to get married and to become housewives are usually spoiled by indulgence, petting, admiration, and this for a quality not at all related to strong character, and therefore vanity of a trivial kind results.

2. Moreover, woman is trained to

emotionality. It may be that she is by nature more emotional than man, but again this can only be known when she has been trained to repress emotional response as a man is trained. If a boy cries or shows fear, he is scolded, and training of one kind or another is instituted to bring about moral and mental hardihood. But if a girl cries, she is consoled by some means and taught that tears are potent weapons, a fact she uses with extraordinary effect later on, especially in dealing with men. If she shows fear, she is protected, sheltered, and given a sort of indulged inferiority.

3. The romantic ideal is constantly held before her in the private counsel of her mother, in the books she reads, in the plays she witnesses, in all the allurements of art. She is to await the lover, the hero; he will take her off with him to dwell in love and happiness forever. All stories, or most of them, end before the heroine develops the neurosis of the housewife. In fact, literature is the worst possible preparation for married life, excepting perhaps the *courtship*. This latter emphasizes a distorted chivalry that makes of woman a petty thing on a pedestal,

out of touch with reality; it is an exciting entrance into what in the majority of cases is a rather monotonous existence.

All these things — vanity, emotionality, romanticism, courtship — are poor training for the home. They hinder even the strongest woman, they are fetters for the more delicate.

In taking up the special types predisposed to the nervousness of the housewife it is to be emphasized that conditions may bring about the neurosis in the normal housewife. Nevertheless, there are groups of women who, because of their make-up or constitution, acquire the neurosis much more easily and much more intensely than do the normal women. They are the types most commonly seen in the hospital clinic or in the private consulting room of the neurologist.

First comes the hyperæsthetic type. One of the chief marks of advancing civilization is an increasing refinement of taste and desire. The fundamental human needs are food, shelter, clothes, sex relations, and companionship. These the savage has as well as his civilized brother, and he finds them not only necessary but agreeable. What we call progress improves the food and the shelter, modifies the clothes, elaborates the sex relations and the code governing companionship. With each step forward the cruder methods become more actively disagreeable, and only the refined methods prove agreeable. In other words, desire keeps pace with improvement, so that although great advances materially have been made, there has been little advance, if any, in contentment. This is because as we progress in refinement little things come to be important, manner becomes more essential than matter, and we get to the hyperæsthetic stage.

Thus the dinner becomes less important than the manner of serving it. In the "highest circles" it is the *savoir faire*, the niceties of conduct, that count more than character. Words become the means of playing with thought rather than the means of expressing it, and thought itself scorns the elemental and fundamental and busies itself with the vagaries of existence.

From another angle, to the hyperæsthetic more and more things have become disagreeable. To the man of simple tastes and simple feelings, only the calamities are disagreeable; to the hyperæsthetic every breeze has a sting, and life is full of pin pricks. "The slings and arrows of outrageous fortune" are multiplied in number, and furthermore the reaction to them is intensified. In the "Arabian Nights" the princess boasts that a rose petal bruises her skin, while her competitor in delicacy is made ill by a fiber of cotton in her silken garments. So with the hyperæsthetic; an unintentional overlooking is reacted to as a deadly insult; the thwarting of any desire robs life of its savor; sounds become noises; a bit of litter, dirt; a little reality, intolerable crudity.

A woman with this temperament is a poor candidate for matrimony unless there goes with it a capacity for adjustment, unusual in this type. Most men have their habitual crudities, their daily lapses, and every home is the theater of a constant struggle with the disagreeable. Intensely pleased by the utmost refinements, these are too uncommon to make up for the shortcomings. The hyperæsthetic woman is constantly the prey of the most deënergizing of emotions, — disgust. "It makes me sick" is not an exaggerated expression of her feeling. And her afflicted household size up the situation with the brief analysis, "Everything makes her nervous." Every one in her household falls under the tyranny of her disposition, mingling their concern with exasperation, their pity with a silent almost subconscious contempt.

Next comes the over-conscientious type. Whatever conscience is, whether implanted by God, or the social code sanctified by training, teaching, and a social nature, there can be no question that, as the Court of Appeals, it does harm as well as good.

There are people whose lack of conscience is back of all manner of crimes, from murder down to careless, slack work; whose cruelty, lust, and selfishness operate unhampered by restraint. On the other hand there are others whose hypertrophied conscience works in one of two directions. If they are zealots, convinced of the righteousness of their own decisions and conclusions, their conscience spurs them on to reforming the world. Since they are more often wrong than right, they become, as it were, a sort of misdirected Providence, raising havoc with the happiness and comfort of others. Whether the conscienceless or those overburdened with this type of conscience have done more harm in the world is perhaps an open question, which I leave to the historians for settlement.

The other type of the overconscientious does definite harm to themselves. This type I have called the "Seekers of Perfection" and it is their affliction that they are miserable with anything less. They are particularly hard on themselves, differing in this wise from the hyperæsthetic. Constantly they examine and reëxamine what they have done. "Is it the best I can do?" "Should I rest now; have I the right to rest?"

Into every moment of enjoyment they obtrude conscience, or rather conscience obtrudes itself. They become wedded to a purpose, and then that purpose becomes a tyrant allowing no escape, even for a brief pleasure, from its chains. Nothing is right that wastes any time; nothing is good but the best. The sense of humor is conspicuously lacking in this type, for one of the main functions of humor is to season effort and straining purpose with proportion.

Should one of these unfortunates be a housewife, then she is continually "picking up", continually pursuing that household Will-o'-the-Wisp, "finishing the work." For it is the nature of housework that it is never finished, no matter how much is done. This overconscientious person, unless she is made of steel springs and resilient rubber, breathlessly chasing this phantom all day and into the night, gives way under the strain, even though she have a dozen servants to help. For to this type each helper is not at all an aid. At once up goes the standard of what is to be done, and each servant becomes an added care, an added responsibility.

"I 'd love to go out with you," wails this housewife, "but there 's something I must finish to-day." The word *must*, self-imposed, becomes the mania of her life, to the open rebellion of her household. The word drives her to the real neglect of her husband, who becomes irritated at her constant and to him needless activity, coupled with her complaints.

"Why don't you rest if you are tired," is his stock remonstrance; "the house looks all right to me."

But it is futile. She becomes irritated, perhaps cries and says, "Just like a man.

It 's clean to you if there are no cobwebs on the walls."

Whereupon the debate closes, but the woman is the more deënergized and the man exasperated at the unreasonableness of women in general and his wife in particular.

It is probably true that woman has more conscience, in so far as detail is concerned, than man. She is more of a lover of order and neatness, more wedded to decorum. Man loves comfort and his interest is more specialized and analytical, and as a rule he hates fussiness.

This hatred of fussiness makes him long for the masculine clubroom, gives him the kind of uneasiness that sends him off on a fishing trip or hunting expedition. Further, and this is of great social importance, many a broken home, many an unexplainable triangle of the Wife, the Husband, and the Other Woman owes its existence, not to the charms of the other woman, but to the overconscientious wife.

The third type predisposed to the neurosis of the housewife is the overemotional woman.

We have already considered the effect of certain types of emotion on health and endurance and may formulate it as follows: Emotion may act as a great bodily disturbance, affecting every organ and every function of the body. What we call nervousness is largely made up of abnormal emotional response, of persistent emotion, of the blocking of energy by emotion.

Now people differ from the very start of life in their response to situations. One baby, if he does not get what he wants, turns his attention to something else, and another will cry for hours or until he gets it. One will manifest anger and strike at being blocked or impeded in his desires, and the other will implore and plead in a baby way for his wish.

In the face of difficulties one man shows fear and worry, another acts hastily and without premeditation, a third flares up in what we call a fighting spirit and seeks to batter down the resistance, and still a fourth becomes very active mentally, calling upon all of his past experience and seeking a definite plan to gain his end.

A loss, a deprivation, plunges one type of person into deepest sorrow, a helpless sorrow, inert and symbolic of the hopeless frustration of love. The same affliction striking at another man's heart makes him deeply and soberly reflective, and out of it there ensues a great philanthropy, a great memorial to his grief. For the one, sorrow has deënergized; for the other it has energized, has raised the efforts to a nobler plane.

Now there are women, and also men, to whom emotion acts like an overdose of a drug. Parenthetically, emotion and certain drugs have very similar effects. No matter how joyous the occasion and how exuberant their joy, a mood may settle into their lives like a fog and obscure everything. This mood may arise from the smallest disappointment; or a sudden vision of possible disaster to one they love may appear before them through some stray mental association. They are at the mercy of every sad memory and of every look into the future.

Preëminently, they are the victims of that form of chronic fear called worry, more aptly named by Fletcher "fearthought." He implied by this name that it was a sort of degenerated "forethought."

If the baby has a cough, then it may have tuberculosis or pneumonia or some disastrous illness, of which death is the commonest ending. How often is the doctor called in by these women and needlessly, and how she does keep his telephone busy! It is true that a cough may be early tuberculosis, but this is the last possibility rather than the first.

If the husband is late, Heaven knows what may have happened. She has visions of him lying dead in some morgue, picked up by the police, or he 's in a hospital terribly injured by an automobile, or, perchance, a robber has sandbagged him and dragged him into a dark alley. If she is a bit jealous, and he is at all attractive, then the disaster lies that way. It does n't matter that his work may be such that he cannot be at home regularly or on schedule; the sinister explanation takes possession of her to the exclusion of the more rational; *she has a sort of affinity for the terrible*. And when her husband comes home, the profound fear in many cases turns sharply and quickly to anger at him. Her distorted sense of responsibility makes him the culprit for her unnecessary fear.

Now it is true that almost every woman has something of this tendency, but it is only the extreme case that I am here depicting. In this extreme form, this type of woman is commonly found among the Jews. The Jewish home reverberates with emotionality and largely through this attitude of the Jewish housewife.

Such a woman is apt to make a slave of her family through their fear of arousing her emotions. How frequently people are chained by their sympathies, how frequently they are impeded in enjoyment by the tyranny of some one else's weakness, would fill one of the biggest chapters in a true history of the human race, — a book that will probably never be written.

Naturally enough, this housewife finds plenty to worry about, to react to, and since these reactions are physical, they have a lowering effect on her energy.

To those familiar with the conception that every emotion, every feeling, needs a discharge, it will seem heretical when I say that the excessive discharge of emotion is harmful. Freud finds the root of most nervous trouble in repressed emotion. That is in part true, but it is also true that excessive emotionality is a high-grade injury, for emotional discharge is habit forming. It becomes habitual to cry too much, to act too angry, to fear too much. The conquest and disciplining of emotion is one of the great objects of training. It has for its goal the supremacy of the noblest organ of the human being, his brain. For proper living there must be emotion — there always will be — but it must be tempered with intelligence if the best good of the individual and the race is to be reached.

The type of woman we must now study is a very modern product, the non-domestic type.

That the great majority of women have a maternal instinct does not nullify the fact that a small number have none whatever. One of the facts of life, not taken into account with a fraction of its true significance and importance, is the variability of the race, the wide range of abilities, instincts, emotions, aspirations, and tastes. A quality is said to be normal when the majority of the group possess it, but it may be utterly lacking in a smaller number who are thereby declared abnormal.

At present, it is normal for woman to be domestic, *i.e.* to yearn for husband, home, and children; to want to be a housewife. Unfortunately, all these yearnings do not hang closely together, and a woman may want a husband and be swept by her own desire and opportunity into matrimony, and yet she may "detest" children, may dislike the housekeeping activities of marriage. The sex and other instincts upon which marriage is based are not always linked with the maternal and home-keeping instincts.

While this has probably always been true, it mattered little in olden days. A woman regarded the home as her destiny and generally had experienced no other life. But as was shown in the first chapter, industry and feminism have given woman a taste of other kinds of life and have developed her individual points of character and abilities. Perhaps she has been the bookkeeper of a large concern; or the private secretary to a man of exciting affairs; or she has been the buyer for some house; or she has dabbled in art or literature; or she has been a factory girl mingling with hundreds of others, working hard, but in a large group; or a saleslady in a department store, — and domestic life is expected of her as if she had been trained for it. In fact, she has been trained away from it.

The novelists delight to tell us of the woman who seeks a career and enters the struggle of her profession and fails. And then there comes, just when her failure is greatest and she is most weepingly feminine, the patient hero, and he holds out his arms, and she slips into them, oh, so joyously! She now has a home, and will be happy — long row of asterisks, and have children; and if it is a movie, a year or more elapses and we are permitted to gaze upon a charming domestic scene.

But alas for reel life as against real life! We are not shown how she yearns for the activities of her old career; we are not shown the feeling she constantly has that she is too good for housekeeping. If she has been fortunate enough to marry a rich and indulgent man, she becomes a dilettante in her work, playing with art or science. If her first vocation was business, she is bored to death by domesticity. But if she marries poverty, she looks on herself as a drudge, and though loyalty and pride may keep her from voicing her regrets, they eat like a canker worm in the bud, — and we have the neurosis of this type of housewife. Or else her experience in business makes her size up her husband more keenly, and we find her rebelling against his failure, criticizing him either openly to the point of domestic disharmony, or inwardly to her own disgust.

It is not meant that all business and professional women, all typists and factory girls are dissatisfied with marriage or develop an abnormal amount of neurosis. Many a girl of this type really loves housekeeping, really loves children, and makes the ideal housewife. Intelligent, clear-eyed, she manages her home like a business. But if independent experience and a non-domestic nature happen to reside in the same woman, then the neurosis appears in full bloom. Against the adulation given to women singers and actresses, against the fancied rewards of literature and business, the domestic lot seems drab to this non-domestic type.

Here the question arises: Is there room in our society for matrimony and a business career? That a large number of exceptional women have found it possible to be mothers, housewives, authors, and singers at one and the same time does not take away from the fact that in the majority of cases such a combination means either a childless marriage or the turning over of an occasional child to servants: it means the abandonment of the home and the living in hotels, except in the few cases where there is wealth and trusty servants. Wherever women who have children are poor and work in factories, there is the greatest infant mortality, there is the greatest amount of juvenile delinquency, and there is the greatest amount of marital difficulty. Our present conception of matrimony demands that woman remains in the home until such time at least as her children are able to care largely for themselves.

In the history of the worst cases of the housewife's neurosis one finds previously existing trouble, though, as I have before this emphasized, the neurosis may develop in the previously normal. This previously existing trouble is the "nervous breakdown" in high school or in college, or in the factory and the office, though it must be said it occurs relatively less often in the latter places than the former. This previous breakdown often appears as the direct result from emotional strain such as an unhappy love affair, or the fear of failure in examinations. It may have followed acute illness, like influenza or pneumonia. But the original temperament was nervous, high-strung, delicate; one learns of an appetite that disappeared easily, a sleep readily disturbed, in short, an easily lowered or obstructed output of energy.

This type of woman, neurotic from her very birth, is often the very best product of our civilization from the standpoint of character and ability, just as the male neurasthenic is often the backbone of progress and advancement. But we are concerned with these questions: "What happens to her in marriage?" "How about her fitness for marriage?"

As to the first question, we may say that all depends on whom and how she marries. For after all a woman does not marry *matrimony*, she marries a *man*, a home, and generally children. And if the neurotic woman marries a devoted, kindly, conscientious man with wealth enough to give her servants in the household and variety in her experiences, she is as reasonably well off as could be expected. She is no worse off than if she had remained single and continued to be a school teacher, social worker, typist, factory hand the rest of her days, — and she has fulfilled more of her desires and functions. But if she marries an unsympathetic, impatient man or a poor one, or a combination, then the first child brings a breakdown that persists, with now and then short periods of betterment, for many years. Then we have the chronic invalid, the despair of a household, the puzzle of the doctors. "Not really sick," say the latter to the discouraged husband, seeking to adjust himself to his wife, "only neurasthenic. All the organs are O. K." To differentiate between a lowered energy and imaginary illness or laziness is a hard task to which this husband is usually unequal. Though some show of duty and kindness remains, love dies in such a household. And the very effort to give sympathy where doubt exists as to the genuineness of the affliction is painful and increases the chasm between wife and husband.

That some of the sweetest marriages result where the wife is of this type does not change the general situation that such a marriage is an increased risk. Should a man knowingly marry such a woman? The question is futile in the overwhelming majority of cases.

He will marry her, is the answer. For the fascinating woman is frequently of this type. Witness the charm of the neuropathic eye with its widely dilated pupil that changes with each emotion, the mobile face, — delicate, with a play of color, red and white, that is charming to look at, but which the grim physician calls "Vasomotor instability." There is nothing neutral about this type; she is either very lovely or a freak.

So all advice in the matter is of little avail. And racially speaking it is good that it is of no avail. I believe firmly that such a woman is more often the mother of high ability than her more placid sister; that something of the delicacy of feeling and intensity of reaction of neurasthenia is a condition of genius. We are too far away from any real knowledge of heredity to advise for or against marriage in the most of cases on this basis, and certainly we must not repeat Lombroso and Nordau's errors and call all variations from stupidity degeneration.

But this does not change the domestic situation of the man who is usually much more concerned with his own comfort than the mathematical possibilities of his offspring being geniuses. Certainly such a woman as the type now considered is not a poor man's wife, for she really needs what only the rich can have, — servants, variety, frequent vacations, and freedom from worry. Now worry cannot be shut out of even the richest home, for illness, old age, and death are grim visitors who ask no man's leave. But poverty and its worries are kept away by wealth, and poverty is perhaps the most persistent tormentor of man.

Essential in the study of "nervousness" is the physical examination, and we here pass to the physically ill housewife.

It is important to remember that the diagnosis of neurasthenia is, properly speaking, what is called by physicians a diagnosis of exclusion. That is to say, after one has excluded all possible illnesses that give rise to symptoms like neurasthenia, then and then only is the diagnosis justified. That is, a woman physically ill, with heart, lung, or kidney disease, or with derangements of the sexual organs, may act precisely like a nervous housewife, — may have pains and aches, changes in mood, loss of control of emotion; in a word may be deënergized.

It is not often enough remembered that bearing children, though a natural process, is hazardous, not only in its immediate dangers but to the future health of the woman. Injuries to the internal and external parts occur with almost every first birth, especially if that birth occurs after twenty-five years of age. Repair of the parts immediately is indicated, but in what percentage of cases is this done? In a very small percentage of cases, I venture to state, not only in my own small experience in this work, but on the statements of men of large experience and high authority.

In this connection I may state that the leading obstetricians believe that the woman of to-day has a harder time in labor than her predecessors. Aside from the more or less mythical stories of the savage women who deliver themselves on the march, there seems to be no reasonable doubt that in an increasing civilization and feminization, woman becomes less able to deliver herself, especially at the first birth.

Why is this? After all, it is a fundamental matter. And moreover it is more often the tennis-playing, horseback-riding, athletic girl who falls short in this respect than the soft-limbed, shrinking, old-fashioned girl. Does a strenuous existence make against easy motherhood? It would seem so; it would seem the more masculine the occupations of woman become, the less able are they to carry out the truly female functions. But this is a digression from our point.

A retroverted uterus, a lacerated perineum, such minor difficulties as flat feet, such major ones as valvular disease of the heart, are causes of ill health to be ruled out before "nervousness" (or its medical equivalents) is to be diagnosed.

It is superfluous to say that we have here briefly considered only a few of the types specially predisposed to difficulty. Moreover men and women do not readily fall into "types." A woman may be hyperæsthetic in one sphere of her tastes and as thick-skinned as a rhinoceros in others. She may squirm with horror if her husband snores in his sleep, but be willing to live in an ugly modern apartment house with a poodle dog for her chief associate. Or the overconscientious woman may expend her energies in chasing the last bit of dirt out of her house but be willing to poison her family with three delicatessen meals a day. The overemotional housewife may flood the household with her tears over trifles but be a very Spartan in the grave emergencies of life. And the neurotic woman, a chronic invalid for housework, may do a dragoon's work for Woman Suffrage. It may be that no man can understand women; it is a fact they do not understand themselves. But in this they are not unlike men.

One might speak of the jealous woman, the selfish woman, the woman envious of her more fortunate sisters, poisoning herself by bitter thoughts. These traits belong to all men and women; they are part of human nature, and they have their great uses as well as their difficulties. Jealousy, selfishness, envy, three of the cardinal sins of the theologian, are likewise three of the great motive forces of mankind. They are important as reactions against life, not as qualities, and we shall so consider them in a later chapter.

Though we have discussed the types predisposed to the nervousness of the housewife, it is a cardinal thesis of this book that great forces of society and the nature of her life situation are mainly responsible. From now on we are face to face with these factors and must consider them frankly and fully.

CHAPTER IV

The Housework and the Home as Factors in the Neurosis

One of the most remarkable of the traits of man is the restless advancement of desire, — and consequently the never-ending search for contentment. What we look upon as a goal is never more than a rung in the ladder, and pressure of one kind or another always forces us on to further weary climbing.

This is based on a great psychological law. If you put your hand in warm water it *feels* warm only for a short time, and you must add still warmer water to renew the stimulus. Or else you must withdraw your hand. The law, which is called the Weber-Fechner Law, applies to all of our desires as well as to our sensations. To appreciate a thing you must lose it; to reach a desire's gratification is to build up new desires.

This is to be emphasized in the case of the

housewife, but with this additional factor: that how one reacts to being a housewife depends on what one expects out of life and housekeeping. If one expects little out of life, aside from being a housewife, then there is contentment. If one expects much, demands much, then the housewife's lot leads to discontent.

What is disagreeable is not a fixed thing, except for pain, hunger, thirst, and death. The disagreeable is the balked desire, the obstructed wish, the offended taste. It is a main thesis of this book that the neurosis of the housewife has a large part of its origin in the increasing desires of women, in their demands for a fuller, more varied life than that afforded by the lot of the housewife. Dissatisfaction, discontent, disgust, discouragement, hidden or open, are part of the factors of the disease. Furthermore there is an increasing sensitiveness of woman to the disagreeable phases of housework.

What are these phases that are attended with difficulty? 1. The status of the house work.

It is an essential phase of housework that as soon as woman can afford it she turns it over to a servant. Furthermore there is greater and greater difficulty in getting servants, which merely means that even the so-called servant class dislikes the work. No amount of argument therefore leads away from the conclusion that housework must be essentially disagreeable, in its completeness. There may be phases of it that are agreeable; some may like the cooking or the sewing, but no one likes these things plus the everlasting picking up; no one likes the dusting, the dishwashing, the clothes washing and ironing, the work that is no sooner finished than it beckons with tyrannical finger to be begun. To say nothing of the care of the children!

I do not class as a housewife the woman who has a cook, two maids, a butler, and a chauffeur, — the woman who merely acts as a sort of manager for the home. I mean the poor woman who has to do all her own work, or nearly all; I mean her somewhat more fortunate sister who has a maid with whom she wrestles to do her share, — who relieves her somewhat but not sufficiently to remove the major part of housewifery. After all, only one woman in ten has any help at all!

It is therefore no exaggeration when I say that though the housewife may be the loveliest and most dignified of women, her work is to a large extent menial. One may arise in indignation at this and speak of the science of housekeeping, of cleanliness, of calories in diet, of child-culture; one may strike a lofty attitude and speak of the Home (capital H), and how it is the corner stone of Society. I can but agree, but I must remind the indignant ones that ditch diggers, garbage collectors, sewer cleaners are the backbone of sanitation and civilization, and yet their occupations are disagreeable.

"Fine words butter no parsnips." There are some rare souls who lend to the humblest tasks the dignity of their natures, but the average person frets and fumes under similar circumstances. In its aims and purposes housekeeping is the highest of professions; in its methods and technique it ranks amongst the lowest of occupations. We must separate results, ideals, aims, and possibilities from methods.

All work at home has the difficulty of the segregation, the isolation of the home. Man, the social animal who needs at least some one to quarrel with, has deliberately isolated his household, somewhat as a squirrel hides nuts, — on a property basis. There has grown up a definite, æsthetic need of privacy; all of modesty and the essential family feeling demand it.

This is good for the man, and perhaps for the children, but not for the woman. Her work is done alone, and at the time her husband comes home and wants to stay there, she would like to get out. Work that is in the main lonely, and work that on the whole leaves the mind free, leads almost inevitably to daydreaming and introspection. These are essentials, in the housework, — monotony, daydreaming, and introspection.

Let us consider monotony and its effects. The need of new stimuli is a paramount need of the human being. Solitary confinement is the worst punishment, so cruel that it is prohibited in some communities. We need the cheerful noises of the world, we need as releasers of our energies the sights, sounds, smells of the earth; we must have the voices and the presence of our fellows, not for education, but for the maintenance of interest in living. For the mind to turn inward on itself is pleasurable only in rare snatches, for short periods of time or for rare and abnormal people. Man's mind loves the outside world but becomes uneasy when confronted by itself.

The human being, whether male or female, housewife or industrial worker, is a seeker of sensations. Without new sensations man falls into boredom or a restless and unhappy state, from which the mind seeks freedom. It is true that one may become a mere seeker of sensations, a restless and fickle pleasure lover who passes from the normal to the abnormal, exotic in his vain search for what is logically impossible, — lasting novelty. Variety however is not the mere spice of life; it is the basis of interest and concentrated purpose as well.

People of course vary greatly in what they regard as variety, and this is often a constitutional matter as well as a matter of education. What is new, striking and interest-provoking to the child has not the same value to the adult; what is boredom to the city man might be of huge interest to the country man. A person trained to a certain type of life, taught to expect certain things, may find no need of other newer things. In other words people accustomed to a wide range of stimuli need a wide range, while people unaccustomed to such a range do not need it.

The most important stimuli are other *persons*, capable of setting into action new thoughts, new emotions, new conduct. We need what Graham Wallas calls "face to face associations of ideas", — ideas called into being by words, moods, and deeds of others.

It is this group of stimuli that the busy housewife conspicuously lacks. "She has no one to talk to," especially in the modern apartment life. It is true she has her children to scold, to discipline, to teach, and to talk *at;* but contact with child minds is not satisfying, has not the flavor of companionship, is not reciprocal in the sense that adult minds are. There therefore results introspection and daydreaming, both of which may be of slight importance to some women but which are distinctly disastrous to others.

If the married life is satisfactory the daydreaming and introspection may be very pleasurable, as they usually are at the beginning of marriage. The young bride dreams of love that does not swerve, of understanding that persists, of success, of riches to come, of children that are lovely and marvelous. And the happy woman also finds her thoughts pleasant ones, and her castles in the air are mere enlargements of her life.

But the dissatisfied woman, the unhappy woman, finds her daydreams pleasant and unpleasant at the same time. She is constantly coming back to reality; reality constantly obtrudes itself into her dreams. The daydreaming is rebelled against as foolish, as puerile, as futile. A struggle takes place in the mind; disloyal and disastrous thoughts creep in which are constantly dismissed but always reappear. The profoundest disgust and deënergization may appear, and fatigue, aches, pains, and weariness of life often results.

One may compare interest to a tonic. How often does one see a little group, who for the time being are not interesting to one another, sit sleepy, tired, bored, yawning, restless. Then a new person enters, a person of importance or of interest. The fatigue disappears like magic, and all are bright, energetic, sparkling. The basis of club life is the monotony of the home; man uses the saloon, the clubroom, the pool room, the street corner, the lodge meeting, as an escape from the unstimulating atmosphere of wife and family, — the hearth. But for the housewife there is usually no escape, though she needs it more than her husband does.

Furthermore the non-domestic type, the woman with especial ability, the woman who has been courted, petted, and sought for before marriage is the one who reacts most to the monotony of the home. There are plenty of women who consider the home a refuge from a world they find more strenuous, more fatiguing than they can stand, or who find in housework a consecration to their ordained duty. Which type is the better woman depends upon the point of view, but it is safe to say that feminism and the industrial world are making it harder and harder for an increasing number of women to settle down to home-keeping.

The housewife is *par excellence* a sedentary creature. She goes to work when she gets up in the morning, within doors. She goes to bed at night, very frequently without having stirred from the home. A great many women, especially those who have no help and have children, find it next to impossible to get out of doors except for such incidental matters as hanging out the clothes or going to the grocery.

It is true that some women so situated get out each day. But they are possessed either of greater energy or skill or else own a less urgent conscience. At least for many women it gets to be a habit to stay in. If there is a moment of leisure, a chair or a couch, and a book or paper, seem the logical way of resting up.

Now sedentary life has several main effects upon health and mood. It tends quite definitely to lower the vigor of the entire organism. Perhaps it is the poor ventilation, perhaps it is the lack of the exercise necessary for good muscle tone that brings about this result. Though the housewife may work hard her muscles need the tone of walking, running, swimming, lifting, that our life for untold centuries before civilization made necessary and pleasurable.

With this sedentary life comes loss of appetite or capricious appetite. Frequently the housewife becomes a nibbler of food, she eats a bite every now and then and never develops a real appetite. Nor is this a female reaction to "food close-at-hand"; watch any male cook, or better still take note of the man of the house on a Sunday. He spends a good part of his day making raids on the ice chest, and it is a frequent enough result to find him "logy" on Monday.

Furthermore, in the household without a servant, the housewife rarely eats her meal in peace and comfort. She jumps up and down from each course, and immediately after the meal she rarely relaxes or rests. The dishes *must* be cleared away and washed, and this keeps from her that peace of mind so necessary for good digestion.

An increasing refinement of taste adds to these difficulties. If the family eat in the dining room, have separate plates for each course, and various utensils for each dish, have snowy linen instead of oilcloth, — then there is more work, more strain, less real comfort. Much of what we call refinement is a cruel burden and entails a grievous waste of human energy and happiness.

An important result of the sedentary life

is constipation. Woman, under the best of circumstances, is more liable to this difficulty than her mate, just as the human being is more liable to it than the four-legged beast. Man's upright position has not been well adjusted by appropriate structures. Child-bearing, lack of vigorous exercise, the corset, and the hustle and bustle of the early morning hours so that regular habits are not formed, bring about a sluggish bowel. Indeed it is a cynicism amongst physicians that the proper definition of woman is "a constipated biped."

While it is a lay habit to ascribe overmuch to constipation, it is also true that it does definite harm. For many people a loaded bowel acts as a mood depressant, as illustrated by the Voltaire story. For others it destroys the appetite and brings about an uneasiness that affects the efficiency. Whether there is a poisoning of the organism, an auto-intoxication, in such a condition is not a settled matter. But the importance of the constipation habit lies chiefly in its effect upon mood and energy, in its relation to neurasthenia.

These factors, the nature of housework, monotony and the results of sedentary life bear with especial weight upon the woman of little means. It is absolutely untrue that nervousness is a disease of wealth. There are cases enough where lack of purpose and lack of routine tasks, as in the case of wealthy women, lead to a rapid demoralization and deënergization. It is also true that the search for pleasure leads to a sterile sort of strenuousness that breaks down the health, as well as inflicting injury on the personality.

Poverty is picturesque only to the outsider. "It's hell to be poor" is the poor man's summary of the situation. There are serious psychical injuries in poverty which will demand our attention later, and still more serious bodily ones. In the case of the housewife, poverty on the physical side means (1) never-ending work; (2) no escape from drudgery and monotony; (3) insufficient convalescence from the injuries of child-bearing; (4) a poor home, badly constructed, badly managed, without conveniences and necessities.

That there are plenty of poor women who bear up well under their burdens is merely a testimony to the inherent vitality of the race. A man would be a wreck morally, physically, and mentally if he coped with his wife's burdens for a month. Either that or the housekeeping would get down to bare essentials. If a man kept such a house, dusting and cleaning would be rare events, meals would become as crude as the needs of life would allow, ironing and linen would be wiped off as non-essential, and the children would run around like so many little animals. In other words an integral part of what we call civilization in the home would disappear.

Perhaps men would reorganize the home. The housekeeper of to-day is only in spots coöperative; her social sense is undeveloped. Men might, and I think likely would, arrange for a group housekeeping such as that which they enjoy in their clubs.

This digression aside, there are debilitating factors in the housewife's lot which need some amplification. We have referred to the insufficient time for convalescence from childbirth. There are *sequelæ* of childbirth, such as varicose veins, flat feet, back strain, that render the victim's life a burden. The rich woman finds it easy to secure rest enough and proper medical attention. But the poor woman, not able to rest, and with recourse either to her overbusy family doctor or to the overburdened, careless, out-patient department of some hospital, drags along with her troubles year in and year out, becomes old before her time, and loses through constant pain and distress the freshness of life.

It is impossible to separate the psychical factors from the physical, largely because there is no separation. One of the aims of a woman's life is to be beautiful, or at least good looking. From her earliest days this is held out to her as a way to praise, flattery, and power. It becomes a cardinal purpose, a goal, even an ideal.

Unlike the purposes of men this goal is attained early, if at all, and then Nature or Life strip it away. The well-to-do woman or the exceptional poor woman may succeed in keeping her figure and her facial beauty for a relatively long time, though by the forties even these have usually given up the struggle. For the poor woman the fading comes early,—household work, bearing children, sedentary life, worry, and a non-appreciative husband bringing about the fatal change.

I doubt if men see their youth slipping

away with the anguish of women. To men, maturity means success, greater proficiency, more achievement, — means purpose-expanding. To women, to whom the main purpose of life is marriage, it means loss of their physical hold on their mate, loss of the longed for and delightful admiration of others; it means substantially the frustration of purpose.

And I have noticed that the very worst cases of neurosis of the housewife come in the early thirties, in women previously beautiful or extraordinarily attractive. They watch the crows'-feet, the fine wrinkles, the fat covering the lines of the neck and body with something of the anguish that the general watches the enemy cutting off his lines of communication or a statesman marks the rise of an implacable rival.

Popular literature, popular art, and popular drama, including in this by a vigorous stretching of the idea the movie, are in a conspiracy against reality. This is of course because of the tyranny of the "Happy Ending." While the happy ending is psychologically and financially necessary, in so far as the publishers, editors, and producers are concerned, what really happens is that the disagreeable phases of life, not being faced, persist. To have a blind side for the disagreeable does not rule it out of existence; in fact, it thus gains in effect.

To say that housekeeping is looked upon essentially as menial, to say that it is monotonous, that it is sedentary, and has the ill effects that arise from these characteristics, is not to deny that it has agreeable phases. It has an agreeable side in its privacy, its individuality, and it fosters certain virtues necessary to civilization. That I do not lay stress on these is because novelist, dramatist, and scenario author, as well as churchman and statesman, have always dwelt on these. The agreeable phases of the housewife's work do not cause her neurosis; it is the disagreeable in her life that do. Or rather it is what any individual housewife finds disagreeable that is of importance, and it is my task to show what these things are, how they work, and finally what to do about it.

CHAPTER V

Reaction to the Disagreeable

A few preliminary words about the disagreeable in the housewife's lot will be of value.

We may divide the things, situations, and happenings of life into three groups, — the agreeable, the indifferent, and the disagreeable. No two men will agree in detail in judging what is agreeable, indifferent, or disagreeable. There are as many different points of view as there are people, and in the end what is one man's meat may literally be another man's poison. There are, however, only a few ways of reacting to what one considers the disagreeable. The agreeable things of life do not cause a neurosis, though they may injure character or impair efficiency. And we may neglect the theoretical indifferent.

1. A disagreeable thing may be so disastrous in our viewpoint as to cause fear.

This fear may be expressed as flight, which is a normal reaction, or it may be expressed by a sort of paralysis of function, as the fainting spell, or the great weakness which makes flight impossible. Fear is a much abused emotion. People speak glibly about taking it out of life, on the ground that it is wholly harmful. "Children must not experience fear; it is wrong, it is immoral; they should grow up in sunshine and gladness, without fear." A whole sect, many minor religions, take this Pollyanna attitude toward reality.

As a matter of fact fear is *a* (I almost said *the*) great motive force of human life. Fear of the elements was the incentive to shelter; fear of starvation started agriculture and the storage of food; fear of disease and death gives medicine its standing; fear of the unknown is the backbone of conservatism, and fear of the rainy day is the source of thrift. Fear of death is not only the basis of religion, but of life insurance as well. Fear of the finger of scorn and the blame of our fellows is the great force in morality. And no amount of attempted unity with God will ever take the place of the injunction to fear Him!

2. While fear then is back of the constructive forces of life it works hand in hand with another emotion that is also greatly disparaged by sentimentalists, — anger. The disagreeable, by balking an instinct, by obstructing a wish or purpose, may arouse anger. The anger may blaze forth in a sudden destructive fury in an effort to remove the obstacle, or it may simmer as a patient sullenness, or it may link itself with thought and become a careful plan to overcome the opposition. It may range all the way from the blow of violence to burning indignation against wrong and injustice; it is the source of the fighting spirit. Without fear, purpose would never be born; without anger in some form or other it would never be fulfilled.

3. But while fear and anger work well in succession, or at different times, when both emotions are awakened by some disagreeable situation or thing, when there is a helpless anger, when the instinct to fight is paralyzed by fear, when doubt arises, then there is deënergization.

Thus a hostile situation, an intensely disagreeable situation, may be met with energy: viz. planning, constructive flight, destructive action, or it may be met with a deënergization, confusion, paralysis, hopeless anger. It may cause an intense inner conflict with high constant emotions, fatigue, incapacity to choose the proper action, and the peculiar agony of doubt.

This last type of reaction is a very common one in the housewife. For the situation is never clear-cut for decision — there is the ideal implanted by training, education, social pressure, and her own desire to live in conformity with this ideal; there is opposing it disgust, anger, weariness, lack of interest that her house duties bring with them. This conflict leads nowhere so far as action is concerned, for she can neither accept nor reject the situation.

This is to say: The human being needs primarily a definite point of view, a definite starting place for his actions. Some belief, some goal, some definite purpose is needed for the rallying of the energy of mind and body. Drifting is intolerable to the acute, active mind bent upon some achievement before death. Man is the only animal keenly aware of his mortality, and consequently he is the only one to fear the passing of time.

This passing of time can be received equably by the one conscious of achievement, or who has some compensation in belief and purpose; it becomes intolerable to those in doubt.

Fundamentally one may say that neurasthenia and the allied diseases which we are here summing up as the nervousness of the housewife are reactions to the disagreeable. The fatigue, pains and aches, changes in mood and emotion are born of this reaction, except in those cases where they arise from definite bodily disease, and even here a vicious circle is established. The weakness and fatigue state, the consciousness of impaired power brought about by sickness, are reacted to in a neurasthenic manner. It is not often enough realized by physicians that a physical defect or a physical injury may be reacted to so as to bring about nervous and mental symptoms; may cause the emotions of fear, hopeless anger, and sorrow; may cause an agony of doubt.

With these few words on types of reactions to the disagreeable let us turn again to the disagreeable factors in our housewife's life which may cause her neurosis.

The child is the central bond of the home and is of course the biological reason for marriage. The maternal instinct has long been recognized as one of the great civilizing factors, the source of much of human sympathy and the gentler emotions. While the beautiful side of the mother-child relationship is well known and cannot be overestimated, the maternal instinct has its fierce, its jealous, its narrow aspect. Love and sympathy for one's own in a competitive world have often as their natural results injustice and hardness for the children of others. While the best type of mother irradiates her love for her own into love for all children, it is not uncommon for women to find their chiefest source of rivalry in the progress and welfare of their children.

Maternal devotion is largely its own reward. The child takes the maternal sacrifices for granted, and after the first few years the interests of parent and child diverge. There is a never-ending struggle between the rising and the receding generations, which is inherent in the nature of things and will always exist wherever the young are free. All the world honors the mother, but few children return in anything like equality the love and sacrifices of their own mother.

Is the maternal instinct waning in intensity in this period of feminization? There have always been some bad, careless, selfish mothers; has their number increased? Probably not, yet the maternal instinct now has competition in the heart of the modern woman. The desire to participate in the world's activity, the desire to learn, to acquire culture, engenders a restless impatience with the closed-in life of the mother-housewife. This interferes with single-minded motherhood, brings about conflict, and so leads to mental and bodily unrest. Of course this interferes little or not at all with some, probably most of the present-day mothers, but is a factor of importance in the lives of many.

The nervous housewife has several difficulties in her relations to her children. These are of importance in understanding her and have been touched on before this, but it will be of advantage to consider them as a group.

We have said that the opinion of obstetricians is that the modern woman has more difficulty in delivering herself than did her ancestress. If this is true (and we may be dealing with the fact that obstetricians are often the ones to see the difficult cases, or that these stand out in their memories) there are several explanations.

First, women marry later than they did. It may be said that the first child is easiest born before the mother is twenty-five years of age, and that from that time on a first child is born with rapidly increasing difficulty. The pelvis, like all the bony-joint structures of the body, loses plasticity with years, and plasticity is the prime need for childbearing. Similarly with the uterus, which is of course a muscular organ, but possesses an elastic force that diminishes as the woman grows older.

Second, the vigor of the uterine contractions upon which the passage of the baby depends is controlled largely by the so-called sympathetic nervous system, though glands throughout the body are very important factors as well. This part of the nervous system and these glands are part of the mechanism of emotion as well as of childbearing, and emotion plays a rôle of importance in childbearing. The modern woman *fears* childbearing as her ancestress did not, partly through greater knowledge, partly through her divided attitude towards life.

Having a harder time in childbearing means a slower convalescence, a need for more rest and care. Then nursing becomes somehow more difficult, more wearing to the mother; she rebels more against it, and yet, knowing its importance, she tries to "keep her milk." It often seems that the more women know about nursing, the less able they are to nurse, that the ignorant slum-dweller who nurses the child each time it cries and drinks beer to furnish milk does better than her enlightened sister who nurses by the clock and drinks milk as a source of her baby's supply.

The feeling of great responsibility for her child's welfare that the modern woman has acquired, as a result of popular education in these matters, undoubtedly saves infants' lives and is therefore worth the price. A secondary result of importance, and one not good, is the added liability to fatigue and breakdown that the mother acquires. This factor we meet again in the next phase of our subject, the education and training of children.

Though the number of children has conspicuously decreased, the care and attention given them has increased in inverse proportion. The woman with six children or more turned over the younger children to the older ones, so that her burden, though heavy, was much less than it may seem. Further, though she loved and cared for them, she knew far less of hygiene than her descendant; she did not try to bring them up in a germless way; and her household activities kept her too busy to allow her to notice each running nose, or each "festering sore." Not having nearly so much knowledge of disease, she had much less fear and was spared this type of deënergization. Her daughter views with alarm each cough and sneeze, has sinister forebodings with each rash; pays an enormous attention to the children's food, and through an increasing attention to detail in her child's life and actions has a greater liability to break under the greater responsibility and conscientiousness.

It must be remembered that the feeling of responsibility and apprehensive attention is not merely "mental." It means fatigue, more disturbance of appetite, and less restful sleep. These are things of great importance in causing nervousness; in fact, they constitute a large part of it.

Perhaps another generation will find that hygiene can be taught without producing fussiness and fear. Certainly popular education has its value, but it has a morbid side that now needs attention. This morbid side is not only bad for the mother but is unqualifiedly bad for the child.

For the child of to-day, the center of the family stage in his attention, is often either spoiled or made neurasthenic by his treatment. Either he is frankly indulged, or else an overcritical attitude is taken toward him. "Bad habits must not be formed" is the actuating motive of the overconscientious parents, for they do not seem to know that the "trial and error" method is the natural way of learning. Children take up one habit after another for the sake of experience and discard them by themselves. For a child to lie, to steal, to fight, to be selfish, to be self-willed is not at all unnatural; for him to have bad table manners and to forget admonition in general and against these manners in particular is his birthright, so to speak.

Yet many a mother of to-day torments her child into a bad introspection and self-consciousness, herself into neurasthenia, and her husband into seething rebellion, because of her desire for perfection, because of her fear that a "bad act" may form into a habit and thence into a vicious character.

Especially is this true of the overæsthetic, overconscientious types described in Chapter III. I have seen women who made the dinner table less a place to eat than a place where a child was pilloried for his manners, — pilloried into sullen, appetiteless state.

So, too, an unfortunate publicity given to child prodigies brought with it for a short time an epidemic of forced intellectual feeding of children, that produced only a precocious neurasthenia as its great result. Similarly the Montessori method of child training which made every woman into a kindergarten teacher did a hundred times more harm than good, despite the merits of the system. That a child needs to experiment with life himself means that it will be a long time before the average mother will know how to help him.

A factor that tends to perplex the mother and hurts the training of the child is her doubt as how "to discipline." Shall it be the old-fashioned corporal punishment of a past generation, the appeal to pain and blame? Shall it be the nowadays emphasized moral suasion, the appeal to conscience and reason? With all the preachers of new methods filling her ear she finds that moral suasion fails in her own child's case, and yet she is afraid of physical punishment.

This is not the place to study child training in any extensive manner, yet it needs be said that praise and blame, pleasure and pain, are the great incentives to conduct. One cannot drive a horse with one rein; neither can one drive a child into social ways, social conformity by one emotion or feeling. Corporal punishment is a necessity, sparingly used but vigorously used when indicated. Of course praise is needed and so is reward.

What is here to be emphasized is that a sense of great responsibility and an overcritical attitude toward the children is a factor of importance in the nervous state of the modern housewife. Increasing knowledge and increasing demand have brought with them bad as well as good results. Here as elsewhere a little knowledge is a dangerous thing, but a more serious difficulty is this, — though fads in training arise that are loudly proclaimed as the only way, there is as yet no real science of character or of character growth.

The tragedy of illness is acute everywhere, and the sick child is in every household. In many cases I have traced the source of the housewife's neurosis to the care and worry furnished by one child. There are truly delicate children who "catch everything", who start off by being difficult to nurse, and who pass from one infection to another until the worried mother suspects disease with every change in the child's color A sick child is often a changed child, changed in all the fundamental emotions, — cranky, capricious, unaffectionate, difficult to care for. A sick child means, except where servants and nurses can be commanded, disturbed sleep, extra work, confinement to the house, heavy expense, and a heightened tension that has as its aftermath, in many cases, collapse. The savor of life seems to go, each day is a throbbing suspense.

With recovery, if the woman can rest, in the majority of cases no marked degree of deënergization follows. But in too many cases rest is not possible, though it is urgently needed. The mother needs the care of convalescence more than does the child.

There is an extraordinary lack of provision for the tired housewife. True there are sanataria galore, with beautiful names, in pretty places, well equipped with nurses and doctors to care for their patients. But these are prohibitive in price, and at the present writing the cheapest place is about forty dollars per week. This rate puts them out of the reach of the great majority who need them.

Moreover, where there are small children and where there is no trusty servant or some kindly relative or friend it seems impossible for the housewife to leave the home. Her husband must work daily for their bread and unless they are willing to turn to the charitable organizations, it is necessary for the housewife to carry on, despite her fatigue. So at the best she gets an hour or two extra rest a day, takes a "little tonic" from the family doctor and gets along with her pains, her aches, and moods as best she can.

But the sick do not always recover. Fortunately, the average human being grieves a while over death, but the life struggle soon absorbs him, and the bereavement itself becomes a memory. But now and then one meets mothers whose griefs and deprivations seem without end. No religion, no philosophy can bring them back into continuity with their lives. They go about in a sorrowful dream, hugging their affliction, resenting any effort to comfort or console; without interest in the daily task or in those whom they should love. They offer the severest problem in readjustment, in reënergization, for they actively resent being helped. Sometimes one believes their grief is an effort to atone for neglect real or fancied, a self-punishment which is not remitted until full atonement has been made.

Aside from the physical difficulties in the bearing and rearing of children, and in addition to the ordinary mental difficulties, such as judging what discipline to use, there are especial problems of some importance. Men vary in character from the saint to the villain, in ability from the genius to the idiot. The children they once were vary as much.

There are children who go through the worst of homes, the worst of environments, the worst of trainings, — and come out pure gold, with characters all the better for the struggle. There are others whom no amount of love, discipline, training, and benefits help; they are despicable from the ordinary viewpoint from the first of life to the last. Some children, adversely situated as to poverty and health, become geniuses, and their reverse is in the poor child whom heredity, early disease, or some freak of nature dooms to feeble-mindedness.

The heart of the mother is in her child; she glories in its progress, and she refuses to see its defects until they glare too brightly to be overlooked. Then she has a heartbreak all the more bitter for her maternal love.

It is the incorrigibly bad child and the mentally deficient child who evoke the severest, most neurasthenic reaction on the part of the housewife. Not only is pride hurt, not only is the expanded self-love injured, but such children are a physical care and burden of such a nature as to outbalance that of three or four normal children.

The bad child, egoistic, undisciplinable,

destructive, and quarrelsome, or the child who cannot be taught honesty, or the one who continually runs away, is an unending source of "nervousness" to his mother. As time goes on and the difficulty is seen to be fundamental, a battle between hostility and love springs up in the mother's breast that plays havoc with her strength and character. The very worst cases of housewife neurosis are seen in such mothers; the most profound interference with mood, emotion, purpose, and energy results.

Similarly, with the mother of the feeble-minded child. At first the child is viewed as a bit slow in walking, talking, in keeping clean, and the mother explains it all away on this ground or that. A previous illness, a fall in which the head was hurt, difficulty with the teething, diet, etc., all receive the blame. Alas! In the course of time the child goes to kindergarten and the terrible report comes back that "the child cannot learn, is clumsy, etc.", and the teacher thinks he should be examined. Then either through the examination or through the pressure of repeated observations mother love yields to the truth and feeble-mindedness is recognized.

There are plenty of women who, with this fact established, adjust themselves, make up their minds to it. But others find that it takes all the pleasure out of their lives, become morbid, and do not enjoy their normal children. For with all due respect to eugenics and statistics I am convinced that the most of feeble-mindedness is accidental or incidental, and not a matter of heredity. Once a mother gets imbued with the notion that the condition is hereditary, she falls into agonies of fear for her other children. In my mind there is a thoroughly reprehensible publicity given to half-baked work in heredity, mental hygiene, and the like that does far more harm than good and interferes with the legitimate work.

There is no offhand solution for the case of the incorrigible boy or girl. Of course the largest number sooner or later reform, sometimes overnight, and in a way to remind one of the religious conversions that James speaks of in his "Varieties of Religious Experiences." So long as a child has a social streak in his make-up, so long as he at least is responsive to the praise and blame of others and understands that he does wrong, so long may one hope for him. But the child to whom the opinion of others seems of no value, who follows his own egoism without check or control by the accepted standard of conduct, by the moral law, by the praise and blame of those near to him, is almost hopeless. Some day intelligence may keep him out of trouble, but by itself it cannot change his nature.

It is not sufficiently realized that while there has been a rise of feminism there has also been a great change in the status of children, a change that makes their care far more difficult than in the past. They have risen from subordinate figures in the household, schooled in absolute obedience, "to be seen and not heard," to the central figures in the household. One of the strangest of revolutions has taken place in America, taken place in almost every household, and without the notice of historians or sociologists. That is because these professional students of humanity have their attention focused on little groups of figures called the leaders, and not nearly enough on that mass which gives the leaders their direction and power.

The age of the child! His development

parallels that of women, in that an individualization has taken place. In the past education and training took notice of the child-group, not of the individual child. But child-culture has taken on new aspects, punishment has been largely superseded, individual study and treatment are the thing. Personality is the aim of education, especial aptitudes are recognized in the various types of schools that have arisen: commercial, industrial, classical; yes, and even schools for the feeble-minded.

All this is admirable, and in another century will bring remarkable results. Even to-day some good has come, but this is largely vitiated by other influences.

Aside from the fact that the attention paid the child often increases his self-importance and makes his wishes more capricious, there are factors that tend to rob him of his naïveté.

These factors are the movies, the newspapers, and the spread of luxurious habits amongst children.

The movies are marvelous agents for the spread of information and misinformation. Because of the natural settings they give to the most absurd and unnatural stories, their essential falsity and unreality is often made the more pernicious. Their possibilities for good are enormous, their actual performance is conspicuously to lower the public taste, to create a habit which discourages earnest reading or intelligent entertainment. For children they act as a stimulant of an unwholesome kind, acquainting them with realistic crime, vice, and vulgarity, giving them a distaste for childlike enjoyment. One sees nowadays altogether too often the satiated child who seeks excitement, the cynical, overwise child filled with the lore of the movies.

In similar fashion the "comic" cartoons of the newspapers have an extraordinary fascination for children. Every child wants to read the funny page, though the funny page is not for childish reading. The humor is coarse, slangy, and distinctly vulgar; very clever frequently and thoroughly enjoyable to those whom it cannot harm.

If the historians of, say, 4500 A.D. were by chance to get hold of a few copies of our newspapers of 1920 they might legitimately conclude that the denizen of this remote period expressed surprise by falling backward out of his shoes, expressed disagreement by striking the other person over the head with a brick or a club; that women were always taller than their mates and usually "beat them up"; that all husbands, especially if elderly, chased after every young and pretty girl. They might conclude that the language of the mass of the people was of such remarkable types as this: "You tell them Casket, I 'm Coffin", or "the Storm and Strife is coming; beat it!"

No one I think enjoys the comic page more than the present writer, — yet it spreads a demoralizing virus amongst children. Of what use is it to teach children good English when the newspaper deliberately teaches them the cheapest slang? Of what use is it to teach them manners and kindliness when the newspaper constantly spreads boorishness and "rough house" conduct? Of what use is it to raise taste when this is injured at the very outset of life by giving bad taste a fascinating attraction?

Throughout the community there is a stir and excitement that is reflecting on the children. There are so many desirable luxuries in the world now, so many revealed by movie and symbolized by the automobile, the cabaret, the increasing vulgarity of the theater (the disappearance of the drama and the omnipresent girl and music show), a restless search for pleasure throughout the community even before the War, have not missed the child.

All these things make the lot of the housewife harder in so far as the training of her children is concerned. She is dealing with a more alert, more sophisticated, more sensuous child, — and one who knows his place and power. The press and the theater both have knowledge of this and a recent witty play dealt with the sins of the children, paraphrasing of course the classic of a bygone day, "Sins of the Fathers." And a wise old gentleman said to his grandson recently, when the lad complained about his mother, "Of course you are right. Every son has a right to be obeyed by his mother."

I am by no means a pessimist. Every forward step has its bad side, but nevertheless is a forward step. It is in the nature of things that we shall never reach a millennium, though we may considerably improve the value and dignity of human life. Democracy has a rôle in the world of great importance, — but the spread of education and opportunity to the mass may make it more difficult for the best ideals and customs to survive in the avalanche of mediocrity that becomes released by the agencies that profit by appealing to the mass. So, too, the rise of the woman and child bring us face to face with new problems, which I think are less difficult problems than those they have superseded and replaced, but which are yet of importance.

And a great problem is this: how to individualize the child and keep from spoiling him; how to give him freedom and pleasure, and keep him from sophistication.

CHAPTER VI

Poverty and Its Psychical Results

In the story of Buddha it is related that it was the shock of learning of the existence of four great evils which aroused his desire to save mankind. These evils were Old Age, Sickness, Death, and Poverty. Theologians and the sentimentalists are unanimous in their praise of poverty, — the theologians because they seek their treasure in heaven, and the sentimentalists because they are incorrigible dodgers of reality, because they cannot endure the existence of evil. But Buddha knew better, and the common sense of mankind has shown itself in the desperate struggle to reach riches.

We have spoken of the part played by the physical disadvantages of poverty in causing the nervousness of the housewife. It is not alleged or affirmed that all poor housewives suffer from the neurosis, — that would be nonsense. But poor food, poor housing, poor clothing, the lack of vacations, the insufficient convalescence from illness and childbirth are not blessings nor do they have anything but a bad effect, an effect traceable in the conditions we are studying.

Furthermore, the woman who does all her own housework, including the cooking, scrubbing, washing, ironing, and the multitudinous details of housekeeping, in addition to the bearing and rearing of children, does more than any human being should do. It is very well to say, "See what the women of a past generation did," but could we look at the thing objectively, we would see that they were little better than slaves. That is the long and short of it, — the Emancipation Proclamation did not include them.

Aside from the physical effects of poverty on the housewife, there are factors of psychical importance that call for a hearing. After all, what is poverty in one age is riches in another; what is poverty for one man is wealth to his neighbor. More than that, what a man considers riches in anticipation is poverty in realization. Here again we deal with the mounting of desire.

The philosophical, contented woman, satisfied with her life even though it is poor, is exempted from one great factor making for breakdown. Contentment is the great shield of the nervous system, the great bulwark against fatigue and obsession. But contentment leads away from achievement, which springs from discontent, from yearning desire. Whether civilization in the sense of our achievements is worth the price paid is a matter upon which the present writer will not presume to pass judgment. Whether it is or not, Mankind is committed to struggle onward, regardless of the result to his peace of mind.

There are two principal psychical injuries with poverty — fear and worry — and we must pass to their consideration as factors in the neuroses of some women.

Worry is chronic fear directed against a life situation, usually anticipated. Man the foreseeing must worry or he dies, — dies of starvation, disease, disaster. It is true that worry may be excessive and directed either against imaginary or inevitable ills; ills that never come, ills that must come, like old age and death.

Men in comfortable places cry "Why worry?" meaning of course that the most of worry is about ills that are never realized. That is true, but the person living just on the brink of disaster, ruined or made dependent on charity by unemployment, a long illness, or any failure of power and strength, cannot be as philosophical as the man fortified by a nice bank account or dividend-paying investments. These well-to-do advisers of the poor remind one of the heroes of ancient fables who, having magic weapons and impenetrable armor, showed no fear in battle. One wonders how much courage they would have had if armed as their foemen were.

For the poor housewife who sees no escape from poverty, whose husband is either a workman or a struggling business man always on the edge of failure, life often seems like a wall closing in, a losing battle without end.

Especially in the middle-aged, in those approaching fifty, does this happen. Aside from the condition produced by "change of life", the so-called involution period, there is a reaction of the "time of life" that is found very commonly. For old age is no longer far off on the horizon; it is close at hand, around the corner, and the looking-glass proclaims its coming. The woman wonders whether her husband will long be able to keep up, — and then "what will become of us?"

To be thrown on the benevolence of children is a sad ending to independent natures, to people of experience. Crudely put, those who have been dependents are now sustainers; those who have been led now guide; the inferiors are the superiors. This is not cynicism, for with the best intentions in the world, if the children are also poor, the care of the parents is a burden that they cannot help showing, sooner or later.

Looking forward to such an ending to the hard work and struggle of a lifetime is part of the worry of poverty, to be classed with the fear of sickness and unemployment.

We may loudly proclaim that one honest man is as good as another, that character is the measure of worth, that success cannot be measured by money. These things are true; the difficulty is not to make people believe it, it is to make people *feel* it. Deeply ingrained in poverty is not alone to be deprived of things desired; more important is the feeling of inferiority that goes with the condition. Only in the Bohemia of the novelists do the poor feel equal to the rich.

One of the fundamental strivings of the human being is the enlargement of the self-feeling, which fundamentally is the wish to be superior, to have the admiration and homage of others. All daydreaming builds this air castle; all ambition has this as its goal. No matter how we disguise it to ourselves and others, the main ends of purpose are power and place. True, we may wish for power and place so as to help others; we may wish them as the result of constructive work and achievement, but the enlargement of self-feeling is the end result of the striving.

To be poor is to be inferior in feeling and applies equally to men and women. Man is a competitive-social animal and competes in everything, from the cleverness and beauty of his children to the excellence of his taste in hats. Money has the advantage of being the symbol of value, of being concrete and definite, and of having the inestimable property of purchasing power.

Now woman is as competitive as her mate. A housewife vies with her neighboring housewives in her clothes, her good looks, her youth, her husband, her children, her home, her housekeeping, her money, — vies with her in folly as well as in wisdom. How much of the extravagance of women (and here is a difficulty to be dealt with later) arises from rivalry only the tongues of women could tell, but it is safe to say that the greater part of it has this origin.

Jealousy and envy are harsh words, yet they stand for traits having a great psychological value. Part of the impetus for effort rises from these feelings, and an incredibly large part. Many a man who bends unremitting in his effort has in mind some man of whose success he is envious, or whose efforts he watches with a jealousy hidden almost from himself.

Upon women these feelings play with devastating force. One may be satisfied with what he has until some one else he knows gets more; that is to say, the causes of most of the dissatisfaction and discontent of the world are envy and jealousy. In many cases it may be a righteous sort of jealousy or envy. A woman, especially because she is a rival of her fellow-woman mainly in small things, becomes acutely miserable when she is outstripped by her neighbor and especially if she is passed by her relatives and intimate friends.

Poverty is especially hard on those intensely ambitious for their children. "They must have the education I did not have; they must have a good time in life which I never had; I don't want them to be poor all their lives like we are." Here is the woman who works herself to the bone, yet is content and well save for her fatigue, if her children respond to her efforts by success in study and by ambitious efforts of their own. But if the struggling mother is so unfortunate as to have drawn in Nature's lottery an unappreciative or a weak-minded child, then the breakdown is tragic.

A poor man is much more apt to be philosophical about poverty for his children than his wife is. He is willing to do what he can for them, but he is more apt to realize what mother love is blind to, — that the average child is unappreciative of the parents' efforts and takes them for granted. The man is more apt to think and say, "Let them stand on their own feet and make their own way; it will do them good." The mother usually longs to spare her children struggle, the father rarely shares this desire except in a mild way.

It may be that there was a time when classes were more fixed, that poverty had less of humiliation and blocked desire than it has at present. That society of all grades is restless with the desire for luxury seems without doubt. How profoundly the psychology of the masses is being altered by education, by the newspaper, the magazine, the movie, the automobile, the fashion changes that make a dress obsolete in a season and above all the department store and the alluring advertisement, no one can hope to even estimate. Modern capitalism reaps great wealth by developing the luxurious, the spendthrift tastes of the poor. It would be a peculiar poetic justice that will make that development into the basis of revolution.

The women of the poor are perhaps even more restless than the men. In fact, it is the women that set the pace in these matters. This is because to woman has fallen the spending of the family funds, a fact of great importance in bringing about discord in the house. As the shopper the poor woman now sees the beautiful things that her ancestors knew nothing of, since there were no department stores in those days. To-day desires are awakened that cannot be fulfilled; she sees other women buying what she can only long for, and an active discontent with her lot appears.

Unphilosophical this, and severely to be deprecated as unworthy of woman. This has been done so often and so effectively (?) by divines, reformers, press, that a mere physician begs leave to remark that it is a natural sequence of the publicity luxury to-day has. *The most successful commercial minds of America are in a conspiracy against the poor Housewife to make her discontented with her lot by increasing her desires;* they are on the job day and night and invade every corner of her world; well, they have succeeded. The divines, etc., who thunder against luxury have no word to say against the department store and the advertising manager.

CHAPTER VII

The Housewife and Her Husband

The husband differs from the wife in this fundamental, — that essentially he is not a house man as she is a house woman. For the man the home is the place where he houses his family and where he rests at night. Here also he spends his leisure time in amount varying with his domesticity. Man writes songs and books about the home, but the woman lives there. Perhaps that is why women have not written sentimental verse about it.

Marriage is variously regarded. "It is a sacrament, a religious sanction, and not to be dissolved by anything but Death." So say a very large group of our people. "It is a contract, governed by law, entered into under certain conditions and to be dissolved only by law." This is the attitude of practically all the governments of the world and rapidly is becoming the dominant point of view. Though the religious combat this conception of marriage, no marriage is legal on religious sanction alone, and the increase of divorce among those claiming to be Catholics is an undisputed fact.

It is only in the last century that the contract side of marriage has been emphasized and become dominant. There has resulted a conflict between the sacramental, sacred point of view and the secular. This conflict, like all other social conflicts, is a part of the inner life of most of the men and women of this generation, influencing their attitude toward marriage, the home, the mate.

For when we say a thing is part of the "spirit of the times" we mean merely that arising as a development of, or a change from, old ideas in the minds of leaders, it has become propagated among the mass. It has become part of their thought, incentive to their action, source of their energies.

Thus sentiment and religion proclaim the sacredness of marriage, its eternal nature, its indissolubility. The law asserts it to be a civil relationship, to be made or unmade by law itself; experience teaches that if it is sacred, then sacredness includes folly, indiscretion, brutality, and crime. Therefore the marriage relationship has become a source of conflict for our times, with opposing champions shouting out their point of view, with books, the movies, the press, the stage, with daily experience adducing cases. The scene of conflict is in the moods and emotions of all of us.

This divided view is particularly the attitude of women and becomes part of the neurosis of the housewife.

After all a woman does not marry an institution; she marries a man with whom she lives, sharing his life. In the natural course of events she becomes the mother of the children to whom he is father. We may dismiss as nonimportant the occasional freak marriage where a man and woman live apart, have no children and meet occasionally,—for obvious purposes. Such a marriage is not only sterile biologically, not only empty of the virtues of marriage, but encounters none of its difficulties.

This intimate individual relationship makes marriage when complete and successful the happiest human experience. Soberly speaking, it is then the flower of existence, satisfying biologically and humanly, giving peace and satisfaction to body and mind. This is the ideal, the "happy ending" at which most romances, novels, plays, and all the daydreams of youth leave us. Warm, cozy, intense domesticity, — where passion is legitimate and love and friendship eternal; where children play around the hearth fire; of which death only is the ending!

This ideal is not realized largely because no ideal is. How often is it closely approximated? Experience says seldom. That implies no reproach against marriage, for we are to judge marriage by the rest of life and not by an ideal. A world in which great wars occur frequently, in which economic conflict is constant, in which sickness and disaster are never absent; where education is occasional, where reason has yet to rule in the larger policies and where folly occupies the high places, — why expect marriage to be more nearly perfect than the life of which it is a part? To be reasonably comfortable and happy in marriage is all we may expect.

What are the difficulties confronting the partners which impede happiness and especially which bring the neurosis of the housewife? For after all we can only examine the field for our own purpose.

We may divide the difficulties as follows from the standpoint of the neurosis of the housewife:

1. Those that arise from the sex relationship itself.

2. Those that arise from conflicts of will, purpose, ideas.

3. Those that arise from the types of husbands.

4. Those that arise from the types of wives. (This has already been considered under the heading Types Predisposed to the Neurosis.)

Before we go on to the consideration of these various factors we must repeat what has been emphasized frequently in this book.

That the change in the status of woman implies difficulty in the marriage relationship. If only *one* will is expected to be dominant in the household, the man's, then there can arise no conflict. If the form of the household is unaltered, but if the woman demands its control or expects equality, then conflict arises. If a woman expects a man to beat her at his pleasure, as has everywhere been the case and still is in some places, if she considers it just, brutality exists only in extremes of violence. If she considers a blow, or even a rough word, an unendurable insult, then brutality arises with the commonest disagreement. In other words, it is comparatively easy to deal with a woman expecting an inferior position, whose individual tastes, wills, ideas, and ideals have never been developed, — the ancient woman; it is very much more difficult to deal with her modern sister.

Happily the day is passing when prudery governed the discussion of sex. Lewdness exists in concealment, suggestion is more provocatory than frankness. The morbidness of men who condemned themselves to celibacy has influenced the world; their fear of sex led to a misguided silence shrouding the wrecks of many a life.

The sex relationship is the basis of marriage. The famous couplet of Rosalind still holds good. The sex instinct (or rather instincts, for coupled with sex-desire is love of beauty, admiration, joy of possession, triumph, etc.) has the unique place of being more regulated by law and custom than any other basic instinct. The law holds that no marriage is consummated until the sex act has taken place, regardless of the words of preacher or State official. The happiness of the first year or years of married life is mostly in its voluptuous bonds, for companionship and comradeship have really not yet arisen. Complementary to this it may be said that much of married misery, especially for the woman, arises from the first marital embrace.

This last is because of the ignorance of men and women, an ignorance wholly due to prudery. The majority of women have been chaste before marriage; the majority of men have not. One would expect therefore knowledge of men, the knowledge of experience. But the experience has been gained with women of a certain type and has not equipped the man to deal with his wife. Though most women know in advance what is expected of them, some are even ignorant of the most elemental facts of sex, and even those who know are unprepared for reality.

Too frequently the man regards himself as a Grand Seigneur with a paramount "Jus Primis Noctis." True, the majority of men are abashed in the presence of innocence and deal gently with it, — but others follow in a repellent way their instinct of possession. Any neurologist of experience has cases where sexual frigidity and neurasthenia in a woman can be traced back to the shock of that all-important first night.

There are savage races in which preparation for marriage is an elementary part of education. We need not follow them into absurdity, but more than the last silly whispered words to bride and groom at the ceremony is necessary. A formal antenuptial enlightenment, frank and expert, is needed by our civilization.

The sex appetite varies as widely as any other human character. Generally speaking, it is believed that sexual passion in women is more episodic than in men, often relating to the menstrual period. In many cases it does not develop as a conscious factor in the woman's life until after marriage, and sometimes not until the first child is born. Certainly desire in the girl is a more generalized, less local, less conscious excitement than it is in the boy who cannot misunderstand his feelings. I think it may safely be said that allowing for the freedom of boys and men, there is native to the male a more urgent passion than to the female. This would be biologically necessary, since upon him devolves not only courtship but the fundamental activity in the sexual act. A passionless woman may have sexual relation, a passionless man cannot.

The disparity in sex desire between a husband and wife may be slight or great. No statistics on the subject will ever be gathered, from the very nature of the facts, but it is safe to say that much more disparity exists than is suspected. And likewise it causes more trouble than is suspected. Where the virility of the mate is inadequate there breeds a subtle dissatisfaction that may corrode domestic happiness and bring about conflict on subjects quite remote from the real issue. Contrariwise, to have relations forced or coaxed on one where desire is lacking brings about disgust, nervous reactions, fatigue of marked nature.

A woman sexually well mated often clings beyond reason to an unworthy mate. Many an inexplicable marriage, many a fantastic loyalty of a good woman to a bad man has its origin where it is least expected, in the sex attachment. Demureness of appearance, refinement of manner, noble ideals are not at all inconsistent with powerful sex feeling. There is no reason why strong, well-controlled passion should be considered anything but a virtue, why the pleasure of the sexual field should, under the social restriction, be regarded as impure.

Too often the latter is the case. Fantastic puritanical ideas often govern both men and women. I have in mind several couples who desired to live continent until such time as children were desired. The biological reasons for the sexual relations seemed to them the only "pure" reasons. Needless to say the resolution broke down under the intimacy of one roof, but meanwhile a conflict was engendered that took some vigorous counsel to dissipate.

This purely occidental idea that sexual pleasure is somehow unworthy is responsible for a disparity of a further kind. There are parts of the physical side of love in which the majority of men need education, though in the well-adjusted married life the proper knowledge comes. Nature has not completely adjusted the sexes to one another; it is the part of the man to bring about that adjustment. This part of the adjustment need not here be detailed; the books of Havelock Ellis are explicit on the matter. Certainly no small share of the difficulties of our housewife result, for it is a law that excitement without gratification brings about nervous instability.

Whether or not the American domestic life is too intimate, too constant, is an important question. For the majority of people, after the first ecstasy of the bridal year, separate rooms might be better than a single chamber occupied together. There are people to whom one bed and one room is symbolic of their close unity, of their joined lives, who find comfort and companionship in the knowledge that their life partner sleeps beside them. Where sexual compatibility or adjustment exists, there is nothing but commendation for this arrangement. Where it does not exist, the separate chambers are better for obvious reasons.

A development of recent times is the rapidly increasing use of what are politely known as birth-control measures. This development is rapidly changing the number of births in the community to a figure below that necessary for the perpetuation of the race. We are not concerned here with the morality or immorality of these measures. Modern woman undoubtedly will continue to take the stand that childbearing should be voluntary, that involuntary motherhood is incompatible with her dignity and status as a person. In this, through the increasing cost of living as well as sympathy with her attitude, she will be backed by her husband. I predict without fear that Church and State will have to adjust themselves to this situation.

The fear of pregnancy has brought about this situation, that many a woman undergoes an agony of symptoms which is only relieved when her monthly function appears. This fear makes the sexual relationship a risk almost outweighing its pleasure. The notoriously "unsafe" character of the contraceptive measures has only diminished this fear, not completely allayed it.

Moreover the contraceptive measures, according to the law that every "solution" breeds new problems, have their place in causing nervousness. Rarely do these measures replace the natural act in satisfaction. Further, some are unable to conquer their repugnance and disgust and some are left excited and unsatisfied. Vasomotor disturbances, neurasthenic symptoms, obsessions, and hysterical phenomena occur in many women as well as in some men. One of the stock questions of the neurologists when examining a married man or woman complaining of neurasthenic symptoms relates to the contraceptive measures used. The channel of discharge of sexual excitement is race old. And this new development blocks that channel. For many persons this is sufficient to deënergize the organism.

At the present time there are two trends in the sex sphere, so far as women are concerned. There is the masculine trend, which is usually called feminism. Women tend to take up the work formerly exclusively belonging to men; they tend to dress more like men, with flat shoes, collars and ties, and tailor-made clothes. They take up the vices of men, — smoking, drinking, — are building up a club life, live in bachelor apartments, call each other by their last names, etc.

Whether with this goes a greater sexual license or not it is difficult to say. The observers best qualified to comment think there has been a decrease in female chastity,

— that the entrance of women in industrial life, the growth of the cities, the increase in automobiles, the greater freedom of women, the dropping of restraint in manner and speech, have brought women's morals somewhat nearer to men's.

The other trend, not entirely separate except for externals, is marked by a hypersexuality, an emphasis of femaleness. This is by far the more common phenomenon and probably more widely spread through society. The dress of women in general is more daring, more designed for sex allurement than for a century past. Women paint and powder in a way that only the demimonde did a generation ago, reminding one of the ladies of the French Court in the eighteenth century. Further, the plays of the day would be called mere burlesque a generation back; the girl and music show has the center of the stage, and the drama in America has almost disappeared. There is an epidemic of magazines that flirt with the risqué; with titles that are sometimes much more clever than their contents.

Such eras have been with us before this, have come and gone. It is doubtful if they ever affected so large a number of people. The excitement of the daily life is increased in a sexual way, and this brings an unrest that reacts on the anchor of the home, the housewife. She too tugs at her moorings; life must be speeded up for her too as well as for the younger and unattached women. She becomes more dissatisfied and therefore more nervous.

Altogether the sexual relationship of modern marriage needs a candid examination. No drastic change is indicated, but education in sexual affairs for men and women is a need. Even the prudish admit the pleasure of the sex-life, and that seems to be their fundamental aversion to it. Most of the advice and injunctions in the past seem to have come from the sexually abnormal. It is time that this was changed; in fact, it is being changed. The danger lies in a swing to extremes, in leaving the fields to those who think reform lies in the abolition of restraint, in the disregard of all social supervision and obligation. Free love is more disastrous if possible than prudery.

CHAPTER VIII

The Housewife and Her Household Conflicts

The problems of life are not all sexual, and in fact even in the relations of men and women there are more important factors. After all, as Spencer pointed out in a marvelous chapter, love itself is a composite of many things, some, of the earth, earthy, and some of the finest stuff our human life holds. The aspirations, the ideals, the yearnings of the girl attach themselves to some man as their fulfillment; the chivalrous feelings, the desire to protect and cherish, the passion for beauty of the man lead to some girl as their goal. There are few for whom the glow and ardor of their young love bring no refinement of their passion; there are few who have not felt a pulsating unity with all that love and live, at least for some ecstatic moments. Something of what James has so beautifully designated as the "aura of infinity that hangs over a young girl" also lingers over the love of men and women.

All the cynics and epigram makers in the world agree that love ends with marriage, and this not only in modern times but even back into those days of the French Court of Love, when Margaret de Valois decided that the lover had more claims than the husband. Romance dies with marriage is the plaint of poet and novelists; the charm of woman disappears with her mystery, with possession. And the typical humorist speaks of the curl papers and kimono of the wife, the snores and unshaven beard of the husband. "Familiarity is the death of passion" is the theme of countless writers who bemoan its passing in the matrimonial state.

How much harm the romantic tales have done to marriage and the sober-satisfying everyday life, no one can estimate, no one can overestimate. Romanticism, which extols sex as the prime and only thing of life, prudery which closes its eyes to it and makes sour faces, need special places in Dante's Inferno. Neither has dealt with reality, — reality, which is satisfying and pleasant unless examined with the prejudices instilled by the hypersexual romance writer and the perverted sexuality of the prude.

Nevertheless that two people brought up entirely differently, and having different attitudes towards love and life, should come into sharp conflict is to be expected. Further, that disillusionment follows after the excitement and heightened expectation of courtship is inevitable. Marriage at the best includes a settlement to routine; it carries with it an adjustment to reality, a getting down to earth that is painful and disappointing to minds fed to expect thrill and passion with each moment.

The idealization of the mate — the man or woman — gives way to a gradually increasing knowledge of imperfection and common clay. Common sense, earnestness of purpose, willingness to adjust, and a sense of humor save the situation and change the love of the engaged period into a more solid, robust affection which gains in durability and wearing quality what it loses in intensity.

Unfortunately, in many cases to a great extent and in all to some extent, there arises dissension natural wherever two human beings meet on anything like equal terms.

In times past (and in many countries at the present time), the patriarchal household prevailed. The Head of the House was the father, a sovereign either stern or indulgent according to his nature. Perhaps his wife ruled him through his love for her, as women have ruled from the beginning of things, but if she did it was not by right but by privilege.

America has changed all that, so say all native and foreign observers. Here the woman rules; here she drags her husband after her like a tail to a kite; here she is mistress and he obeys, though nominally still head of the household. All the humorists emphasize this, and the novelist depicts it as the common situation. The husband is represented as yoked to the wheel of his wife's whims, tyrannized over by the one he works for.

This is surely a gross exaggeration, though it furnishes excellent material for satire. The man still makes the main conditions of life for both; his name is taken, his work sustains the household, his purse supplies the means of existence, his industrial business situation determines the residence, his social standing is theirs. This does not prevent him from being "henpecked" in many cases, but on the whole it assures his superior status.

Nevertheless it is true that the American woman of whatever origin has a will of her own as no other woman has. Since the expression of will is one of the chief sources of human pleasures, one of the chief, most persistent activities, man and wife enter into a contest for supremacy in the household. It may be settled quietly and without even recognizing its existence, on the common plan that the woman shall have charge of the home and the man of his business; it may rage with violence over the fundamental as well as the trivial things of home. After all, it is not the importance of a thing that determines the size of the row it may raise; men have killed each other over a nickel because defeat over even this trifle was intolerable.

What are the chief sources of conflict? For to name them all would be simply to name every possible source of difference of opinion that exists. Let us take as an example Extravagance.

This is a new development. In the former

days the bulk of purchases was made by the husband, in whose hands the purse strings were tightly clutched. With the growth of the cities and industry, the development of the department store and rise of shopping as an institution, the man gave place to his wife largely because industry would not let him off during the daytime. So the housewife disbursed most of the funds of her home, — and there arose one of the fiercest and most persistent of domestic conflicts.

Despite the fact that most American husbands turn over their purses to their wives, they still regard the money as their own. The desire to "get ahead" is an insistent one, returning with redoubled force after each expenditure. He finds his entire income gone each week or month, or finds less left than he expected. "Where does it all go?" is his cry; "Must we spend as much as we do?" "How do people get along who get less than we do?"

To this his wife has the answer, "We must have *this*, and we *must* have that. We must live as our neighbors do."

Here is the keynote to the situation. There has been a democratization of society of this nature; there has been a spread throughout the community of aristocratic tastes. The woman of even the poor and the middle classes must have her spring and autumn suits, her dresses for summer, her summer and winter hats. Her husband too must change his clothes with each shift of the season. For this the enterprise of the clothing trade, the splendid display of the department stores are responsible, awakening desire and dissatisfaction.

While the man accuses the woman of extravagance, he is as guilty as she. He too spends money freely, — on his cigars and cigarettes, on every edition of the newspapers, on the shine which he might easily apply himself, on a thousand and one nickels that become a muckle. The American is lavish, hates to stint, detests being a "piker", says, "Oh, what 's the difference; it will all be the same in a hundred years," but kicks himself mentally afterwards.

Meanwhile he quarrels with his wife, who really is extravagant. In this battle the man wins, even if he loses, for he rarely broods over the defeat. But it brings about a sense of tension in his wife; it brings about a disunion in her heart, because she wants to please her husband, and at the same time she wants to "keep up" with her neighbors and friends. And who sets the pace for her, for all of her group; who establishes the standard of expenditure? Not the thrifty, saving woman, not the one who mends her clothes and makes her own hats, but the extravagant woman, the rich woman perhaps of recently acquired wealth who cares little for a dollar. Against her better judgment the woman of the house enters a race with no ending and becomes intensely dissatisfied, while her husband becomes desperate over the bills.

This disunion in her spirit does what all such disunions do, — it predisposes her to a breakdown. It makes the housework harder; it makes the relations with her husband more difficult. It takes away pleasure and leaves discontent and doubt, — the mother-stuff of nervousness.

While most American husbands are generous, there are enough stingy ones to set off their neighbors. To these men the goal of life is the accumulation of money, as indeed it is with the majority. But to them that goal is to be reached by saving every penny, by denying themselves and theirs all expenditures beyond the necessities.

The woman who marries such a man is humiliated to the quick by his attitude. That a man values a dollar more than he does her wish is an insult to the sensitive woman. There ensues either a never-ending battle with estrangement, or else a beaten woman (for the stingy are stubborn) accepts her lot with a broken spirit, sad and deënergized. Or perhaps, it should be added, a third result may come about; the woman accepts the man's ideal of life and joins with him in their scrimping campaign. With this agreement life goes on happily enough.

It is not of course meant that all or a great majority of American women have difficulties with their husbands over money. But I have in mind several patients who would be happy if this never-ending problem were settled. The struggle "gets on the nerves" of the partners; they say things they regret and act with an impatience that has its root in fatigue.

This difficulty over money and its spending gets worse in the late thirties and early forties, for it is then the man realizes with a startled spirit that he is getting into middle age, that sickness and death are taking their toll of his friends, and that he has not got on. The sense of failure irritates him, depresses him. He finds that he and his wife look at the money situation from a different angle.

"If you loved me," says she, "you would see things a little more my way."

"If you loved me," says he, "you would not act to worry me so."

Here in the year 1920, the high cost of living is becoming the strain of life. Capital and Labor are at each other's throats; men cry "profiteer" at those whom good fortune and callous conscience have allowed to take advantage of the world crisis. The air is filled with the whispers that a crash is coming, though the theaters are crowded, the automobile manufacturers are burdened with orders, and the shops brazenly display the most gorgeous and extravagant gowns. That the marital happiness of the country is threatened by this I do not see recorded in any of the discussions on the subject. Yet this phase of the high cost of living is perhaps its most important result.

The housewife's money difficulties are not confined to the question of expenditure. For there is a factor not consciously put forward but evident upon a little probing.

If a woman remains poor, either actually or relatively, she always knows some man with whom she was familiar in her youth who became rich, or she has a woman friend whose husband has become successful. A subtle sort of regret for her marriage may and does arise in many a woman, a subtle disrespect for her husband because of his failure. The husband becomes aware of her decreased admiration, and he is hurt in his tenderest place, his pride. One of the worst cases of neurasthenia I have seen in a housewife arose in such a woman, who struggled between loyalty and contempt until exhausted. For she came of a successful family, she had married against their counsel and her husband, though good, was an entire failure financially. Measuring men by their success, she found her lowered position almost unendurable but was too proud to acknowledge her error. Out of this division in feelings came a complete deënergization.

Whether or not such a housewife deserves

any sympathy in her trouble, it is certain she presents a problem to every one connected with her.

While money and expenditure afford a fertile field from which nervousness arises, there are others of importance.

Disagreement and disunion, conflict, arise over the training and care of the children. Here the different reactions of a man and woman — *e.g.* to a boy's pranks — causes a taking of sides that is disastrous to the peace of the family. Usually the American father believes his wife is too fussy about his son's manners and derelictions, secretly or otherwise he is quite pleased when his son develops into a "regular" boy, — tough, mischievous, and aggressive. But sometimes it is the overstern father who arouses the mother's concern for the child. If a frank quarrel results, no definite neurotic symptoms follow. It is when the woman fears to side against the husband and watches the discipline with vexation and inner agony that she lowers her energy in the way repeatedly described.

Next perhaps to actual disloyalty women feel most the cessation of the attentions, courtesies, and remembrances of their unmarried life. Women expect this to happen and usually they forgive it in the man who devotes himself to his family, struggles for a livelihood or better, and helps in the care of the children. It is the hyperæsthetic type of housewife spoken of previously who weighs against her husband's devotion a minor dereliction in courtesy.

For it is too common in women to let a momentary neglect or absent-minded discourtesy outweigh a lifetime of devotion. This is part of a feminine devotion to manner and form, of which men are, comparatively speaking, innocent.

Aside from this phase of woman's character there are men who either rapidly or gradually resume after marriage their bachelor freedom, to the neglect of their wives. Though for some time after marriage they give up their "freedom" to play consort and escort, sooner or later they sink back into finding their recreation with their male friends, — at club, lodge, saloon, pool room, etc. When night comes they are restless. At first one excuse or another takes them out, later they break boldly from the domestic ties and only occasionally and under protest do they stay at home or escort the housewife to church, visiting, or the theater.

(It needs be said at this point that in America married life often proceeds too far in the domestication of the man, in his complete separation from male companionship, in a never-broken companionship between man and wife. This is distinctly unhealthy for the man, for he requires in his recreation the sense of freedom from restraint that he can have only in masculine company; where the difficult attitude of chivalry can be discarded for an equality and a frankness impossible even with his wife.)

The housewife, thus left alone, though wounded, may adjust herself. She may build up a companionship for herself in church or amongst her neighbors; she may leave her husband and get a divorce; she may become unfaithful on the basis that turn about is fair play; she may devote herself with greater zeal to her home and children and build up a serene life against odds.

But often she does none of these things. Hurt in her pride, she struggles to gain back her husband. Tears and reproaches fail, sickness sometimes succeeds. If she is childless she becomes obsessed with the belief that a child would hold her husband home. If she is failing in the freshness of her beauty she makes a pathetic effort to hold her indifferent mate through cosmetics and beauty specialists. Without the courage and character to make or break the situation she falls into a feeling of inferiority from which originates her headaches, her feelings of unreality, her loss of enthusiasm, her depressed mind and body.

This type of woman, dependent upon the love and affection of her husband for her health and strength, mental and physical, is the type that woman's education and training, at least in the past, have tended to make. She has not been taught, she has not the power, to stand in life alone; she is the clinging vine to the man's oak, she is the traditional woman. She is happy and well with the right man, but Heaven help her if the marriage ceremony links her with a philanderer! For she has been taught to accept as true and right that mischievous couplet:

> Love is of man's life a thing apart,
> 'T is woman's whole existence.

We need for our womanhood a braver standpoint than that, one more firmly based, less apt to bring failure and disaster. For neither man nor woman should love be the whole existence. It should be a fundamental purpose interwoven with other purposes.

Fortunately one source of domestic difficulty will soon pass from America, — alcoholism. Politicians and theorizers may speak of the blow to individual liberty and satirically prophesy that soon coffee and tobacco will be legislated out also. They need to read Gilbert Chesterton and learn that though "a tree grows upward it stops growing and never reaches the sky." To see, as I do, the almost complete absence of delirium tremens from the emergency and city hospitals, where once every Sunday morning found a dozen or two of raving men; to witness the disappearance of alcoholic insanity from our asylums, where once it constituted fifteen per cent of the male admissions; to see cruelty to children drop to one tenth of its former incidence; to know that former drunkards are steadily at work to the joy of their wives and the good of their own souls, — this is to make one bitterly impatient with the chatter about the "joy and pleasure of life gone," etc. etc., that has become the stock-in-trade of the stage and the press. Though alcoholism did not cause all poverty, it stupefied men's minds so that they permitted much preventable poverty; though it did not cause all immorality, a few drinks often sent a good man to the brothel; and what is more, many of the brothel inmates endured their life largely because of the stupefying use of alcohol.

No one knows the evil of alcohol more than the poor housewife. Of course the woman brought up to believe that drunkenness was to be expected in a man — and who often drank with him — was a victim without severe mental anguish, though her whole life was ruined by drink. But for the refined woman who married a clean, clever young fellow only to have him come home some day reeking of liquor, — silly, obscene, helpless, — *her* contact with John Barleycorn took the joy and sweetness from her life. She often adjusted herself, but in many cases adjustment failed, and a chronic state of bruised and tingling nervousness resulted.

A future generation will not consider it possible that the people of a century that saw the use of wireless, the airship, radium, and the X-ray could think intoxication with its literal poisoning funny, could make a stock humorous situation out of it, and could regard the habit-forming drug that caused it a necessity.

After all is said and done, the fiercest domestic conflicts arise out of the inherent childishness of men and women. Pride and the unwillingness to concede personal error, overtender egoism, bossiness, and rebellion against it, petty jealousies and stubbornness, — these are the basic elements in discord. Children quarrel about trifles, children are unreasonably jealous, children fight for leadership and seek constantly to enlarge their ego as against their comrades. Any one who watches two five-year-olds for an hour will observe a dozen conflicts. So with many husbands and wives.

Unreason, petty jealousy, stubbornness over trifles, bossiness (not leadership), overready temper and overready tears, — these cause more domestic difficulty than alcohol and unfaithfulness put together. The education of American women is certainly not tending to eradicate these defects, which are not necessarily feminine, from her character. In the domestic struggle the man has the major faults as his burden; the woman has a host of minor ones. She claims equality for her virtues yet demands a tender consideration for her weaknesses.

Dealing with petty annoyances, disagreeing over petty matters, with her mind engrossed in her disillusions and grievances, many a woman finds her disagreeables a burden too much for her "nerves." That a philosophy of life would save her is of course obvious, but this is a matter which we shall deal with later.

CHAPTER IX

The Symptoms as Weapons against the Husband

Throughout life, two great trends may be picked out of the intricacy of human motives and conduct. The one is (or may be called) the Will to Power, the other the Will to Fellowship. The will to power is the desire to conquer the environment, to lead one's fellows, to accumulate wealth (power), to write a great book (influence or power), to become a religious leader (power), to be successful in any department of human effort. In every group, from a few tots playing in the grass to gray-headed statesmen deciding a world's destinies, there is a struggle of these wills to power. In the children's group this takes the trivial (to us) form as to who shall be "policeman" or "teacher", in the statesmen it takes the "weighty" form as to which river shall form a boundary line and which group of capitalists shall exploit this or that benighted country. The will to power includes all trends which inflate the ego, — love of admiration, pride, reluctance to admit error, desire for beauty, lust for possession, cruelty, even philanthropy, which in many cases is the good man's desire for power over the lives of his fellows.

Side by side with this group of instincts and purposes, interplaying and interweaving with it, modifying it and being modified by it, is the group we call the will to fellowship. This is the social sense, the need of other's good will, the desire to help, sympathy, love, friendly feeling, self-sacrifice, sense of fair play, all the impulses that are essentially maternal and paternal, devotion to the interests of others. This will to fellowship permeates all groups, little and big, old and young, and is the cement stuff of life, holding society together.

There are those who find no difference between the *egoism* of the will to power and the *altruism* of the will to fellowship. They assert that if egoism is given a wider range, so that the ego includes others, you have altruism, which therefore is only an egoism of a larger ego. However true this may be logically, for all practical purposes we may separate these two trends in human nature.

In each individual there goes on from cradle to grave a struggle between the will to power and the will to fellowship. The teaching of morality is largely the government, the subordination of the will to power; the teaching of success and achievement is largely the discovery of means by which it is to be gained. However we may disguise it to ourselves, power is what we mainly seek, though we may call our goal knowledge, science, benevolence, invention, government, money.

Without the will to fellowship the will to power is tyranny, harshness, cruelty, autocracy, and men hate the possessor of such a character. Without the will to power, the will to fellowship is sterile, futile, and the owner becomes lost in a world of striving people who brush him aside. The two must mingle. And a curious thing becomes evident in the life of men, which in itself is simple enough to understand. When men who have been ruthless, concentrated on success, specialists in the will to power, reach their goal, they often turn to the thwarted will to fellowship for real satisfaction in life, become philanthropists, world benefactors, etc. On the other hand those who start out with ideals of altruism and service, specialists in the will to fellowship, generally lose enthusiasm for this and turn slowly, half reluctantly, to the will for power. In life's cycle it is common to see the egotist turn philanthropist, and the altruist, the idealist, lose faith and become an egotist.

How does this apply to the nervous housewife? Simply this, that there are various ways of seeking power, of gaining one's ends.

There is first the method of force, directly applied. The strong man disdains subtlety, persuasion, sweeps opposition aside. "Might is right" is his motto; he beats down opposition by fist, by sword, by thundering voice, or look. Men who use this method are little troubled by codes; they follow the primitive line of direct attack.

There is second the method of strategy, the disguise of purpose, the disguise of means. The effort is to shift the attention of the opponent to another place and then to walk off with the prize. "Possession is nine points of the law" say these folk. And a straight line is *not* the shortest way for strategy. Or exchange with your opponent, give what *seems* valuable for what *is* valuable and then fall back on the adage, "A fair exchange is no robbery."

Third, there is persuasion. Here, by stirring your opponent into friendliness, he talks matters over, he aligns his interest with yours. Compromise is the keynote, coöperation the watchword. "'T is folly to fight, we both lose by battle; whose is the gain?"

Fourth is the method of the weak, to gain an end through weakness, through arousing sympathy, by parading grief, by awakening the discomfort of unpleasant emotion in an opponent who is of course not an implacable enemy. This has been woman's weapon from time immemorial; tears and sobs are her sword and gun. Unable to cope with man on an equal plane, through his superior physical strength, his intrenched social and legal position, she took advantage of her beauty and desirability, of his love; if that failed, she fell back on her grief and sorrow by which to plague him into submission, into yielding. Children use this weapon constantly; they cry for a thing and develop symptoms in the face of some disagreeable event, such as a threatened punishment. In their day-dreams the idea of dying to punish their cruel parents is a favorite one.

This appeal to the conscience of the stronger through a demonstration of weakness may be called "Will to Power through Weakness." It has long been known to women that a man is usually helpless in the presence of woman's tears, if it is apparent that something he has done has brought about the deluge. And in the case of some housewives, certain similarities between tears and the symptoms appear that show that in these cases, at least, the symptoms of nervousness appear as a substitute for tears in the marital conflict.

Not that this is a deliberate and fully conscious process, nor that it causes the symptoms. On the contrary, it is a use for them!

Such a conclusion of course is not to be reached in those cases where the symptoms arise out of sickness of some kind, or where they follow long and arduous household tasks. But every one knows that the woman who gets sick, has a nervous headache, weakness, a loss of appetite, or becomes blue as soon as she loses in some domestic argument, or when her will is crossed; these symptoms persist until the exasperated but helpless husband yields the point at issue. Then recovery takes place almost at once.

In some of the severer cases of neurasthenia in women such a mechanism can be traced. There is a definite relation between the onset of the attacks and some domestic difficulty, and though the recovery does not take place at once, an adjustment in favor of the wife causes the condition to turn soon for the better.

I do not claim that the above is an original discovery. True, the medical men have not formulated it in their textbooks, but every experienced practitioner knows it to occur. And the humorists and the satirists of the daily press use the theme every day. The favorite point is that the brutal husband is forced to his knees through the disabilities of his wife, and that cure takes place when— he gets her the bonnet or dress she wants, when the trip to Florida is ordered, etc. etc.

Discreditable to women? Discreditable to

those women who use it? Men would do the same in the face of superior force. In the battle of wills that goes on in life the weak must use different weapons than the strong. Doubtless the women of another day, trained otherwise than our present-day women and having a different relationship to men, will abandon, at least in larger part, the weapons of weakness. Wherever women work with men on a plane of equality they ask no favors and resort to no tears. They play the game as men do, as "good sports." But where the relationship is the one-sided affair of matrimony, a certain type uses her tears, her aches and pains, her moods, and her failings to gain her point.

CHAPTER X

Histories of Some Severe Cases

The cases that follow represent mainly the severe types of nervousness in the housewife. To every case that comes to the neurologist there are a hundred that explain their symptoms as "stomach trouble", "backache", etc., who remain well enough to carry on, and who think their pains and aches inevitably wrapped with the lot of woman.

It will be seen, upon reading these cases, that a rather pessimistic attitude is taken toward some of them. It would be nice to present a series of cases all of which recovered, and it would be easy to do that by picking the cases. Such a series would be optimistic in its trend; it would however have the small demerit of being false to life. Though the majority of women suffering from nervousness may be relieved or cured, a number cannot be essentially benefited.

Some of them have temperaments utterly incompatible with matrimony, others have husbands of the incorrigible type, others have life situations to change which would make it necessary to change society. Therefore in these cases all a doctor can do is to *relieve symptoms*, relieve some of the distress and rest content with that.

I am essentially neither pessimist nor optimist in the presentation of these cases, nor do I seek to present the man or woman's case with prejudice. In life a realistic attitude is the best, for if we were to remove much of the sentimental self-deception at present so prevalent, huge reforms would occur almost overnight. Sentimentality decorates and disguises all kinds of horridness and makes us feel kindly toward evil. Strip it away, and we would immediately break down the evil.

There is always this danger in presenting "cases" to a lay public, that symptoms are suggested to a great many people. How deeply suggestible the mass of people can be is only appreciated when one sees the result of public health lectures and books. Many persons tend to develop all the symptoms they hear of, from pains and aches to mental failure. Even in the medical schools this is so, and every medical teacher is consulted each year by students who feel sure they have the diseases he has described.

So in presenting the following cases symptoms will be largely omitted. What will be presented is history and to a certain extent treatment. That part of treatment which is strictly medical can only be indicated.

It may be said that in obtaining the intimate history of a woman a difficulty is met with in the natural reluctance to telling what often seems to the patient painful and unnecessary details. To some people it seems inconceivable that fears, pains and aches, sleeplessness, etc., can arise out of difficulties like the monotony of housework, temperament, or troubles with the husband. Furthermore, though some women understand well enough the source of their conflicts, they are ashamed to tell and rest mainly on the surface of their symptoms. To obtain the truth it is necessary to see the patient over and over again, to get somewhat closer to her. This is especially easy to do after the physician has to a certain extent relieved the patient. In other words, except in the cases where the woman is quite prepared to tell of her intimate difficulties, it is best to go slowly from the medical to the social-psychological point of view.

Case I. The overworked, under-rested type of housewife.

Mrs. A. J., thirty years old, is a woman of American birth and ancestry. Her parents were poor, her father being a mechanic in a factory town of Massachusetts. She had several brothers and sisters, all of whom reached maturity and most of whom married.

Before marriage she was a salesgirl in a department store, worked fairly hard for rather small pay, but was strong, jolly, liked dancing and amusements, liked men and had her girl friends.

At the age of twenty-two she married a mechanic of twenty-four, a good, sober, steady man, devoted to her and very domestic. Unfortunately he was not very well for some time following a pneumonia in the third year of their marriage. They drew upon all their savings and fell seriously in debt. This meant borrowing and scrimping for several years, — a fact which had great bearing on the wife's illness later.

They had three children, born the twelfth month, the third year, and the fourth year after marriage. After the first child the mother was very well, nursed the baby successfully, and the little family flourished. Then came the unfortunate illness of the husband, which threw him out of work for six months, during which time they lived on an allowance from his union, his savings, and finally ran into debt. This greatly grieved the man and depressed the woman, but both bore up well under it until the birth of the second child, when their circumstances forced them to move to a poorer apartment. The wife was delivered by a dispensary physician, who did his duty well but allowed the woman, who protested she felt well, to get up and care for her husband and baby much earlier than she should have done.

The nursing of this baby was more difficult. The mother's breasts did not seem to be nearly as active as in the previous case. The baby cried a great deal and needed attention a good part of the night. The husband was unable to help as he had previously done and the fatigue of the care of child and man brought a condition where the woman was tired all the time. Still she bore up well, though when the summer came she greatly missed the little two weeks' vacation that she and her husband had yearly taken together from the days of their courtship.

The husband recovered, but his strength came back very slowly. He went to work as soon as possible but worked only part time for six months. At night he came home utterly exhausted and could not help his wife at all.

During the next year both children were sick, first with scarlet fever and then with whooping cough. The mother did most of the nursing, though by this time the father was able to help and did. The necessary expenses so depleted the family treasury that when the summer came neither could afford to go away.

Both noticed that the mother was getting more irritable than was natural to her. She went out very seldom and her youthful good looks had largely been replaced by a sharp-featured anxiety. Though she carried on faithfully she had to rest frequently and at night tossed restlessly, though greatly fatigued.

She became pregnant again, much to her dismay and to the great regret of her husband. At times she thought of abortion, but only in a desperate way. The last few months of her term were in the very hot months of the year and she was very uncomfortable. However, she was delivered safely, got up in a week to help in the care of her other two children and to get the house into shape again. Her milk was fairly plentiful, despite her fatigue and "jumpy nerves." Unfortunately at this time, when they had accumulated a little surplus and she was looking forward to better clothes for her family and more comforts, the plant at which her husband was employed suspended operations because of some "high finance" mix-up. Coming at this time, the news struck terror into her heart; she broke down, became "hysterical", *i.e.* had an emotional outburst. This passed away, but now she was sleepless, had no appetite, complained of headache and great fatigue.

Though she was assured that the plant would reopen soon (in fact it soon did), she made little progress. That she was suffering from a psychoneurosis was evident;

what remained was to bring about treatment.

This was done by enlisting a development of recent days, — the Social Service agencies. Out of the old-time charity has come a fine successor, social service; out of the amateurish, self-consciously gracious and sweet Lady Bountiful has come the social worker. Unfortunately social service has not yet dropped the name "Charity", perhaps has not been able to do so, largely because the well-to-do from whom the money must come like to think of themselves as charitable, rather than as the beneficiaries of the social system giving to the unfortunates of that system.

Let me say one more word about social service and the social worker, though I feel that a volume of praise would be more fitting. The social worker has become an indispensable part of the hospital organization, an investigator to bring in facts, a social adjuster to bring about cure. For a hospital to be without a social service department is to confess itself behind the times and inefficient.

Briefly, this is what was done for this family.

Their prejudices against social aid were removed by emphasizing that they were not recipients of charity. The husband was allowed to pay, or arrange to pay, for a six weeks' stay in the country for the mother and the new baby. The home for this purpose was found by the agency and was that of a kindly elderly couple who took the woman into their hearts as well as over their threshold. The social worker arranged with a nursing organization to send a worker to the man's house each day to clean up the home while the children stayed in a nursery. One way or another the husband and children were made comfortable, and the wife came back from her stay, made over, eager to get back to her work.

It is obvious that in such a case as this the physician is largely diagnostician and director, the actual treatment consisting in getting a selfish and inert social system to help out one of its victims. That a sick man should be left to sink or swim, though he has previously been industrious and a good member of society, is injustice and social inefficiency. That a woman, under such circumstances, should be left with the entire burden on her hands is part of the stupidity and cruelty of society.

How avert such a thing? For one thing do away with the name "Charity" in relief work, — and find some system by which industry will adequately care for its victims. What system will do that? I fear it may be called socialistic to suggest that some of the fifteen billions spent last year on luxuries might better be shifted to social amelioration. The record in automobile production would be more pleasing if it did not mean a shift from real social wealth to individual luxury.

Case II. The over-rich, purposeless woman.

This type is of course the direct opposite of the woman in Case I and represents the kind of woman usually held up as most commonly afflicted with "nervousness." "If she really had something to do," say the critics, "she would not be nervous."

This is fundamentally true of her, though not true of the majority of women whom we have discussed. It seems difficult to believe that hard work and worry may bring the same results as idleness and dissatisfaction, but it is true that both deënergize the organism, the body and mind, and so are kindred evils. What's the matter with the poor is their poverty, while the matter with the rich is their wealth.

Mrs. A. De L. is of middle-class people whose parents lived beyond their means and educated their only daughter to do the same. Here is one of the anomalies of life: bitterly aware of their folly, the extravagant and struggling deliberately push their children into the same road. Mrs. De L. learned early that the chief objects of life in general were to keep up appearances and kill time; that as a means to success a woman must get a rich husband and keep beautiful. Being an intelligent girl and pretty she managed to get the rich husband, — and settled down to the rich housewife's neurosis.

Her husband was old-fashioned despite his rather new wealth, and they had two children, — a large modern American family. Though he allowed her to have servants he insisted that she manage their household, which she did with rebellion for a short time, and then rather quickly broke away from it by turning over the household to a housekeeper. This brought about the silent disapproval of her husband, who let her "have her own way", as he said, "because it 's the fashion nowadays."

She became a seeker of pleasure and sensation, drifting from one type of amusement to the other in an intricately mixed co-operation and rivalry with members of her set. She followed every fad that infests staid old Boston, from the esoteric to the erotic. She became an accomplished dancer, ran her own car, followed the races, went to art exhibitions, subscribed to courses of lectures of which she would attend the first, dabbled in new religions, became enthusiastic about social work for a month or two, — and became a professional at bridge. Summers she rested by chasing pleasure and flirting with male *habitués* of fashionable summer resorts; part of the winter she recuperated at Palm Beach, where she vied for the leadership of her set with her dearest enemy.

Her husband financed all her ventures with a disillusioned shrug of his shoulders. As she entered the thirties she became intensely dissatisfied with herself and her life, tried to get back to active supervision of her home but found herself in the way, though her children were greatly pleased and her husband sceptical. The need of excitement and change persisted; gradually an intense boredom came over her. Her interest in life was dulled and she began a mad search for some sensation that would take away the distressing self-reproach and dissatisfaction. Shortly after this she lost the power to sleep and had a host of symptoms which need not be detailed here.

The medical treatment was first to restore sleep. I may say that this is a first step of great importance, no matter how the sleeplessness originates. For even if an idea or a disturbing emotion is its cause, the sleeplessness may become a habit and needs energetic attention.

With this done, attention was paid to the social situation, the life habits. It was pointed out that all the philosophies of life were based on simple living and work, and that all the wise men from the beginning of the written word to our own times have shown the futility of seeking pleasure. It was shown that to be a sensation seeker was to court boredom and apathy, and that these had deënergized her.

For interest in the world is the great source

of energy and the great marshaler of energy. From the child bored by lack of playmates, who brightens up at the sight of a woolly little dog, to the old and vigorous man who makes the mistake of resigning from work, this function of interest can be shown.

She was advised to get a fundamental, nonegoistic purpose, one that would rally both her emotions and her intelligence into service. Finally she was told bluntly that on these steps depended her health and that from now on any breakdown would be merely a confession of failure in reasonableness and purpose.

That she improved greatly and came back to her normal health I know. Whether she continued to remain well and how far she followed the advice given I cannot say. From the earliest time to this, necessity has been the main spur to purpose, and probably the lure of social competition drew the lady back to her old life. Experience, though the best teacher, seems to have the same need of repetition that all teaching does.

Case III. The physically sick woman who displays nervousness.

Though this is one of the most important

of the types of nervous housewife the subject is essentially medical. We shall therefore not detail any case, but it is wise to re-emphasize some facts.

There are bodily diseases of which the early and predominant symptoms are classed as "nervousness." Hyperthyroidism, or Graves' Disease, a condition in which there is overactivity of the thyroid gland and which is particularly prevalent among young women, is one of those diseases. In this condition excitability, irritability, emotional outbursts, fatigue, restlessness, digestive disorders, vasomotor disorders, appear before the characteristic symptoms do.

Neuro-syphilis is another such disease. This is an involvement of the nervous system by syphilis. One of the tragedies that distresses even hardened doctors is to find some fine woman who has acquired neuro-syphilis through her husband, though he himself may remain well. In the early stages this disease not only has neurasthenic symptoms but is very responsive to treatment, and thus the early diagnosis is of great importance.

What is known as reflex nervousness arises as a result of minor local conditions, such as astigmatism and other eye conditions, trouble with the nose and throat and trouble with the organs of generation. The latter is especially important in any consideration of nervousness in the housewife, particularly in the woman who has borne children. Frequently too the existence of hemorrhoids, resulting from constipation, acts to increase the irritability of a woman who is perhaps too modest to consult a physician regarding such trouble. Where such modesty exists (and it is found in the very women one would be apt to think were the very last to be swayed by it), then a competent woman physician should be consulted. With good women physicians and surgeons in every large community there is no reason for reluctance to be examined on the part of any woman.

Further details are not necessary. Enough has been said to emphasize the fact that the nervousness of the housewife is first a medical problem and then a social-psychological one.

Case IV. A case presenting bad hygiene as the essential factor.

Bad hygiene is something more than exposure to bad air, poor food, contaminated water, etc. It includes habits and times of eating, attention to the bowels, outdoor exercise, sleep, and in the marital state it includes the sexual indulgence.

The housewife under consideration, Mrs. T. F., aged twenty-eight, married five years, two children, complained mainly of headache, occasional dizziness, great irritability, and fatigue, so that quarrels with her husband were very common, though there seemed nothing to quarrel about. The family was not rich, but lived in a comfortable apartment; there were no serious financial burdens, the children were reasonably healthy and good, and the closest questioning revealed the husband as a kindly man who never took the initiative in quarrels but who was never able to keep silent under provocation. The couple was still in love and there seemed to be no essential incompatibility.

Questioned as to her habits, Mrs. F. said she did all her own housework except the washing and ironing and scrubbing. She had a little girl three times a week to take the baby out. Before marriage she had been a stenographer, but never earned high pay and had no love for her work. In fact she gave it up with relief and found housework with its disagreeable features much more to her taste than business. She had been of a placid, pleasant temperament and could not understand the change in her.

Since all this did not explain her symptoms, closer inquiry was made into her habits. She arose with her husband at seven-thirty, prepared his breakfast, sent the oldest child off to kindergarten and then had her own breakfast, which usually consisted of toast and coffee. At noon she had a very small piece of meat or an egg and a few potatoes with tea. At night she ate sparingly of the dinner, which usually was meat, potatoes, another vegetable, and a dessert. Her husband here stated that she ate at this meal less than the boy of four and a half.

Comparing her buxom figure with the diet a discrepancy was at once apparent. She then confessed with shame that she was a constant nibbler, eating a bit of this or that every half hour or so, and consequently never had an appetite. The food thus nibbled usually was either spicy or sweet, and she consumed quite a bit of candy. Her bowels moved infrequently and she always needed laxatives. In her spare time she felt rather "logy", rarely went out, except now and then at night with her husband, and spent her leisure hours on the couch reading or nibbling.

This in itself would have quite explained much of her trouble. It has been pointed out that body and mind are not separable; that mental functions are based on the bodily functions, and that mood may rest on no more exalted cause then the condition of the bowels. But a more intimate questioning revealed sexual habits which are easily drifted into by people of an amorous turn of character and who are really fond of one another. These both husband and wife frankly said they had not meant to speak of, but with their disclosure it was evident that a good deal of importance was to be attached to them.

The correction of the life habits was of course the fundamental need. The young woman was instructed in detail as to diet, the care of the bowels and outdoor exercise. Since she was in perfect condition except for stoutness she could easily look for recovery, and as an added incentive the restoration of youthful good looks was held out as certain.

The sexual life was frankly discussed, and necessary restrictions were imposed. Both the husband and wife agreed willingly to the changes ordered and promised faithfully to carry out instructions.

The patient made a splendid recovery and very rapidly. Here was a deënergization dependent solely upon the sedentary life of the housewife and upon ignorance of sex hygiene. Here were quarreling and impending marital disaster removed by attention to details in living. Here was a complete proof that not only does a sound mind need a sound body, but that a sound marriage needs one as well.

Case V. The hyperæsthetic woman.

Mrs. J. F. is twenty-seven years of age. She was born in the United States, of middling well-to-do people. Her father was a gruff, hearty man, not in the least bit finicky, who really despised manners and the like, though he was conventional enough in his own way. Her mother was an old-fashioned housewife, fond of her home and family, in fact perhaps more attached to the former than the latter. She hated servants and got along without them (except for a day woman) until she became rather too old to do the work.

J.'s sister and two brothers were duplicates of the parents, — hearty, stolid, and remarkably plain looking. J., the younger sister, though not the youngest in the family, was as different from her family as if she had sprung from another stock. She was slender, very pretty, with a quick, alert mind which jumped at conclusions, because labored analysis fatigued it. Above all, from the very start of life she was sensitive to a degree that perplexed her family, who were however intensely sympathetic because they adored her. This adoration arose from the fact that J. was brighter and prettier than most of her friends, and that her cleverness in many directions — music, writing, talking, handiwork — was the talk of their little group.

This sensitiveness arose from two main factors. First, an egoism fostered by the worship of her friends and the leadership of her group, — an egoism which led her to regard as a sort of insult anything disagreeable. Accustomed to praise, the least criticism implied or outspoken cut like a knife; accustomed to being waited upon, she resented physical discomfort of the slightest kind. Second, there must also have been an actual physical sensitiveness to sights, sounds, smells, tastes, etc. that made her perceive what others failed to notice. This led to an artistry manifested by her nice work in music and decoration and also by an excessive displeasure at the inartistic.

With this training, experience, and natural temperament she should have married a rich collector of art products, who would have added her to his collection and cherished her as his most fragile possession. Instead, through the working of that strange law of contraries by which Nature strikes averages between extremes, she fell in love with a hulk of a man whose ideas on art were limited to calling a picture "pretty", who loved sports and the pleasures of the table, and whose business motto was "Beat the other guy to it." A successful man, troubled with few subtleties either of approach or conscience, he viewed the marriage relationship in the old-fashioned way and the new American indulgence. A man's wife was to be given all the clothes she wanted, servants to help run the home, ought to bear two or three children, and love her indulgent husband. As for any real intimacy, he knew nothing of it. Kindly, self-indulgent, wife-indulgent, child-indulgent, ruthless in business, he may stand as something America has produced without any effort.

From the very first night J.'s world was shattered. We need not enter into details in this matter, but a woman of this type needs finesse in the initiation into marriage more than at any other time. Cave-man style outraged her every fiber, and the man was dumbfounded at her reaction. Though he tried to make amends his very effort and lack of understanding complicated matters.

Aside from this matter, which in the course of time became adjusted, so that though she rebelled desire arose in her, she found herself at odds with her husband's tastes and conduct in little things. Though his table manners were good enough, the gusto of his eating annoyed her and took away her own appetite. When they went to a play together the coarse jokes and the plainly sensuous aroused his enthusiasm. He lacked subtlety and could not understand the "finer" things of life. As he grew settled in matrimony, which he enjoyed in spite of her nerves (which he took for granted as like a woman), he grew stouter and this irritated and jarred her.

She finally realized she no longer loved him. It is doubtful if she realized this before the birth of her first and only child. She lacked maternal feeling and rebelled with a bitter rebellion against the distortion of her figure that came with the pregnancy. The nursing ordered by the doctor and expected by all around her nearly drove her "wild", she said, for she felt like a "cow", a "female." Indeed she reacted bitterly against the femaleness that marriage forced on her and hated the essential maleness of her husband. Her emotional reaction against nursing took away her milk, and finally the disgusted family doctor ordered the baby weaned and he was turned over to a servant.

She went back to her own life, determined to become a housewife, to see if she could not love her husband and her home. But everything he did irritated her, and everything in the house made her feel as in a "luxurious cage." Yet she was by no means a feminist; she detested "noisy suffragettes", thought women doctors and lawyers ridiculous, and had been brought up to regard marriage as indissoluble.

Gradually out of the conflict, the chilling fear that she had made a mistake which could not be rectified, the constant irritation and annoyances, the revolt against her own sex feeling and her life situation, arose the neurosis. It took the form mainly of sudden unaccountable fears with faint dizzy feelings. The family physician on the aside told me that it was "just a case of a damn fool woman with everybody too good to her."

What constitutes a "damn fool" will include every person in the world, according to some one else. It seemed obvious to me that J. was not meant by nature to be a housewife or any kind of wife. Matrimonially she was a misfit, unless she met some man of a type like herself, though I doubt if any man could have pleased her. I doubt if her over-exacting taste would not rebel against the animal in life itself. For though the animal of life is essentially as fine as the human, certain types find it impossible to acknowledge it in themselves.

At any rate I advised separation for a time, — six months at least. I told the woman her reaction to her husband was abnormal and finicky. She answered that she knew this but could not conceive of any change. We discussed the matter in all its ramifications, and though she and her husband agreed to the separation, I knew that he was determined to hold her to her contract. She improved somewhat but I believe that such a temperament is incompatible with marriage, at least to such a man. The outlook is therefore a poor one.

Case VI. The over-conscientious housewife, — the seeker of perfection.

The woman whose history is to be discussed comes from a family of New England stock, *i.e.* the Anglo-Saxon strain modified by New England climate, diet, history, religion, and tradition into a distinct type. This type, often traditionally conservative and often extraordinarily radical, has this prevailing trait, — standards of right and wrong are set up somehow or other, and a remarkably consistent effort is made to maintain these inflexibly. However, the hyperconscientious are not peculiarly New England alone; I have met Jewish women, Italians, French, Irish, and Negroes who showed the same loyalty to a self-imposed ideal.

This lady, Mrs. F. B., thirty-five years

of age, with three children, was brought by her husband against her will. He declared that both she and he were on the verge of nervous prostration; that unless something was done he would start beating her, this last of course representing a type of humorous desperation that usually has a wish concealed in it. She was "worn to a frazzle", always tired, sleepless, of capricious appetite, irritable, complaining, and yet absolutely refused to see a physician. She had taken tonics by the gallon, been overhauled by a dozen specialists, all of whom say, "nothing wrong of any importance — yet she is a wreck and I am getting to be one."

Her husband was a jolly looking personage from the Middle West, in a small business which kept his family comfortably. He looked domestic and admitted he was, which his wife corroborated. Evidently he was exasperated and worried as he gave the history of the case, with his wife now and then putting in a word: "Now, John, you are stretching things there; don't believe him, Doctor; not so bad as all that," etc.

She was a slender person, rather dowdily dressed as compared with her husband, with garments quite a little behind the prevailing mode. Her hair was unbecomingly put up, and it was evident that she disdained cosmetics of any kind, even the innocent rice powder. Her hands were quite unmanicured, though they were, of course, clean and neat. The hat was the simplest straw, home trimmed and neat, but a mere "lid" compared to the creations most women of her class were at the time wearing. That clothes were meant to be ornamental as well as useful was an attitude she completely rejected.

It turned out that life to her was an eternal housekeeping, — from the beginning of the day to the end she was on the job. Though she had a maid this did not relieve her much, for she constantly fretted and fumed over the maid's slackness. Everything had to be spotless *all the time;* she could not bear the disordered moments of bedtime, of the early morning hours, of wash day, of meal preparation, of the children's room, etc. She was obsessed by cleanliness and order, and her exasperated efforts, her reaction to any untidiness kept her husband and children bound in a fear like her own, though they rebelled and scolded her for it.

"She 's always after the children," said her husband. "She is crazy about them, but she has got them so they don't dare call their soul their own. They don't bring their playmates into the house largely because they know that mother, though she wants children to play, goes after them picking up and cleaning."

This restlessness in the presence of disorder was accompanied by the effort to eradicate all vices, all discourtesies, all errors in manners from the children. She feared "bad habits" as she feared immorality. She thought that any rudeness might grow into a habit, must be broken early; any selfish manifestation might be the beginning of a gross selfishness, any lying or pilfering might be the beginning of a career of crime.

Here one might hold forth on the necessity for trial and error in children's lives. They want to try things, they form little habits for a day, a week, a month which they discard after a while; they try out words and phrases, playing with them and then pass on to a new experiment. They are insatiable seekers of experience, untiring in their quest for experiment, — and they learn thereby. Not every mickle grows into a muckle, and the supplanting of habits, the discarding of them as unsatisfactory, is as marked a phenomenon as the formation of habits.

So our patient allowed nothing for imperfections, experimental stages, developing tastes in her children. She was, however, hardest on herself, self-critical, scolded herself constantly because her house was never perfect, her work never done. She never had time to go out; she had become a veritable slave to a conscience that prodded her every time she read a book, took a nap, or went to a picture show.

It was not at first obvious either to her or her husband that her own ideal of cleanliness and perfection was responsible for her neurasthenia. If her "stomach was out of order ought she not have some stomach remedy; if her nerves were out of order would the doctor not prescribe a nerve tonic or a sedative?" The idea of a medicine for everything is still strong in the community and especially amongst dwellers in small towns, and represents a latent belief in magic.

In addition to such medicines as I thought the situation demanded, and to such advice as bore on her attitude to work and play, I hinted that dressing more fashionably might be of value. For the poorly dressed always have a feeling of inferiority in the presence of the better dressed, and this feeling is seriously disagreeable. To raise the ego-feeling one must remove feelings of inferiority, and here was a relatively simple situation. This woman really cared about clothes, admired them, but had got it into her head early in life that it was sinful to be vain about one's looks. Though she had discarded the sin idea the notion lingered in the form of "unworthy of a sensible woman", "extravagance", etc. As she was painfully self-conscious in the presence of others as a result, this was a hidden reason for sticking to her home.

This woman had a really fine intelligence, wanted to be well and made a gallant effort to change her attitude. In this she succeeded, became as she put it more "careless of her things and more careful of her people." Of course one cannot expect her ever to be anything but a fine housekeeper but she manages to be comfortable and has conquered an over-zealous conscience.

CHAPTER XI

Other Typical Cases

Case VII. The ambitious woman discontented with her husband's ability.

In the American marriage relationship the woman makes the home and the man makes the fortune. In some countries the wife is an active business partner. This is notably true in France, among the Jews in Russia, and many immigrant races in the United States. The wife may even take the leadership if her superiority clearly shows up. Perhaps the American method works well enough in a majority of cases, but there are superior women yoked to inferior men who finally despair of their husband's advancement, and who, as the phrase goes, ought to be "wearing the trousers" themselves.

Mrs. D. J., thirty-nine years old, married fourteen years, two children, had excellent health before marriage. Her family, originally poor, had been characterized by great success. Her brothers occupy important places in the business world and are wealthy. One of her sisters is married to a man who is successful in law, and the other sister is an executive in a department store.

Before marriage Mrs. J. was in her brother's business, and at the time of her marriage earned a comfortable salary. She married a man who inherited a small business, and when they married she was enthusiastic over the prospects of this business. But unfortunately her husband never followed her plans; he listened impatiently and went ahead in his own way. As a result of his conservatism they had not advanced at all financially. Though they were not poor as compared with the mass of people, they were poor as compared with her brothers and brother-in-law.

In addition to the exasperation over her husband's attitude toward her counsel (which was approved by her brothers), she developed a disrespect for him, a feeling that he was to be a failure and a certain contempt crept into her attitude. Against this she struggled, but as the time went on the feeling became almost too strong to be disguised and caused many quarrels. It is probable that if her own brothers and sisters had not done so well her feeling toward her husband would not have reached the proportions it did, for she became envious of the good things they enjoyed and to a certain extent resented her sisters-in-law's attitude toward her husband and herself as poor. The part futile jealousy and envy play in life will not be underestimated by those who will candidly view their own feelings when they hear of the success of those who are near them. One of the reasons that ostentation and bragging are in such disfavor is because of the unpleasant envy and jealousy they tend involuntarily to arouse.

With disrespect came a distaste for sexual relations, and here was a complicating factor of a decisive kind. She developed a disgust that brought about hysterical symptoms and finally she took refuge in refusal to live as a wife. This aroused her husband's anger and suspicions; he accused her of infidelity and had her watched. The disunion proceeded to the point of actual separation, and she then passed into an acute nervous condition, marked by fear, restlessness, sleeplessness, and fatigue.

The analysis of this patient's reactions was difficult and as much surmised as acknowledged. With her breakdown her husband's affection immediately revived and his solicitude and tenderness awoke her old feeling, together with remorse for her attitude towards his lack of business success. It was obvious to me in the few times I saw her that she was working out her own salvation and that no one's assistance was necessary after she understood herself. Intelligence is a prime essential to cure in such cases, — an ignorant or unintelligent woman with such reactions cannot be dealt with. Gradually her intelligence took command, new resolves and purposes grew out of her illness, and it may confidently be said that though she never will be a phlegmatic observer of her husband's struggles she has conquered her old criticism and hostility.

Case VII. The nondomestic type and the mother-in-law.

That there is a nondomestic type of woman to-day is due to the rise of feminism and the fascination of industry. Where a woman has once been in the swirl of business, has been part of an organization and has tasted financial success, settling down may be possible, but is much more difficult than to the woman of past generations. Such a woman probably has never cooked a meal, or mended a stocking, or washed dishes, — and she has been financially independent. For love of a man she gives all this up, and even under the best of circumstances has her agonies of doubt and rebellion.

Mrs. A. O'L. had added to these difficulties the mother-in-law question. She was an orphan when she married, and was the private secretary of a business man who because she was efficient and intelligent and loyal gave her a good salary. She knew his affairs almost as well as he did and was treated with deference by the entire organization.

She married at twenty-six a man entirely worthy of her love, a junior official in a bank, looked on as a rising man, of excellent personal habits and attractive physique. She resigned her position gladly and went into the home he furnished, prepared to become a good wife and mother.

Unfortunately there already was a woman in the house, Mr. O'L.'s mother. She was a good lady, a widow, and had made her home with the son for some years. She was a capable, efficient housewife, with a narrow range of sympathies, and with no ambitions. There arose at once the almost inevitable conflict between mother-in-law and daughter-in-law.

Some day perhaps we shall know just why the husband's mother and his wife get along best under two roofs, though the husband's father presents no great difficulties. Perhaps in the attachment of a mother to a son there is something of jealousy, which is aroused against the other woman; perhaps women are more fiercely critical of women than men are. Perhaps the mother, if she has a good son, is apt to think no woman good enough for him, and if she is not consulted in the choosing is apt to feel resentment. Perhaps to be supplanted as mistress of the household or to fear such supplantment is the basic factor. At any rate, the old Chinese pictorial representation of trouble as "two women under one roof" represents the state in most cases where mother-in-law and daughter-in-law live together.

The senior Mrs. O'L. began a campaign of criticism against the younger woman. There was enough to find fault with, since the wife was absolutely inexperienced. But she was entirely new to hostile criticism, and it impeded her learning. Furthermore, she was not inclined to try all of the mother-in-law's suggestions; she had books which took diametrically the opposite point of view in some matters. There were some warm discussions between the ladies, and a spirit of rebellion took possession of the wife. This was emphasized by the fact that she found herself very lonely and longed secretly for the hum and stir of the office; for the deference and the courtesy she had received there. Further, the distracted husband, in his rôles of husband and son, found himself displeasing both his wife and his mother. He tried to get the girl to subordinate herself, since he knew that this would be impossible for his mother. To this his wife acceded, but was greatly hurt in her pride, felt somehow lowered, and became quite depressed. The house seemed "like a prison with a cross old woman as a jailer", as she expressed it.

Another factor of importance needs some space. The bridal year needs seclusion, on account of a normal voluptuousness that attends it. No outsider should witness the embraces and the kisses; no outsider should be present to impede the tender talks and the outlet of feeling. It sometimes happens that the elderly have a reaction against all love-making; having outlived it they are disgusted thereby, they find it animal like, though indeed it is the lyric poetry of life. So it was in this case; the mother was a third party where three is more than a crowd, and she was a critical, disgusted third party. The young woman found herself taking a similar attitude to the love-making, found herself inhibiting her emotions and had a furtive feeling of being spied on.

The previously strong, energetic girl quickly broke down. Physical strength and energy may come entirely from a united spirit; a disunited spirit lowers the physical endurance remarkably. She became disloyal to matrimony, rebelled against housework, and yet loved her husband intensely. A prey to conflicting ideas and emotions, she fell into a circular thinking and feeling, where depressed thoughts cannot be dismissed and depressed energy follows depressed mood. Prominent in the symptoms were headache, sleeplessness, etc., for which the neurologist was consulted.

How to remedy this situation was to tax the wisdom of a Solomon. It probably would have remained insoluble, had not the statement I made that the main element in the difficulty was the mother-in-law *vs.* daughter-in-law situation come to the ears of the old lady. Conscientious and well-meaning, that lady announced her determination to take up her residence with a married daughter who already had a well-organized household, and whose husband was a favorite of the mother's. Despite the mother-in-law joke of the humorists, the mother-in-law is far more friendly to a daughter's husband than to a son's wife.

This solved part of my patient's problem. There remained the adjustment to domestic life. This was hard, and though in part successful, it was delayed by the sterility of the marriage. The husband and wife agreed that pending a child she might well become active again in the larger world. Though the best place would have been her old work, pride and convention stood in the way, and so she entered upon more or less amateurish social work. Finally, perhaps as an unconsciously humorous compensation for her own troubles, she became an ardent and thoroughly efficient secretary to a league of housewives that aimed at better conditions. This work took up her time except for the supervising of a servant, and this nondomestic arrangement worked well since she had no children.

Case VIII. The childless, neglected woman.

It happened that two of the severest cases I have seen occurred, one in a Jewish woman and the other in a young Irish woman, with such an identity of symptoms and social domestic background that either case might have been interchanged for the other without any appreciable difference. The factors in the cases might simply be summarized as childlessness, anxiety, neglect, and loneliness, and in each case the main symptoms were anxiety, attacks of cardiac symptoms, fatigue, and sleeplessness.

The young Jewish woman, thirty years of age, had been married since the age of twenty. Before marriage she worked in the needle trades, was well and strong and had no knowledge of any particular nervous or mental disease in her family. She married a man of twenty-four, who had also been in the tailoring business and had branched out in a small way in business. This business required him to go to work at about seven-thirty in the morning and he finished at nine-thirty in the evening. In the earlier years of their marriage he came home rather promptly at the end of his long day and the pair were quite happy.

At about the third year after marriage the woman became quite alarmed at her continued sterility. She commenced to consult physicians and in the course of the next three years underwent three operations with no result. She began to brood over this, especially since about this time her husband began to show a decided lack of interest in the home. He would come home at twelve and later, and she found that he was playing cards, — in fact had become a confirmed gambler. When she first discovered this, she became greatly worried; made a trip to New York where his people lived and induced them to bring pressure to bear on him for reform. This they did, with the result that for about six months he remained away from cards and gave more attention to his wife.

The reform lasted only for a short period and then the husband plunged deeper into gaming than ever, and there were periods of three and four days at a stretch when he would not return home at all. At such times the lonely wife, who still loved her husband, fell into a perturbed and agitated frame of mind, the worse because she confided her difficulties to no one. When he would return, shamefaced and repentant, she would reproach him bitterly and this would bring about renewed attention, gifts, etc., for a week or so, — and then backsliding. Finally even the brief spasmodic reforms grew less common, her reproaches were answered hotly or listened to with indifference, and she became "practically a widow" except for the occasions when the sexual feeling mastered them both.

The neurosis in this case approached almost an insanity. The dwelling alone, the desperate obsessive desire for a child to bring back his love and attentions and to satisfy her own maternal instinct, the pain the sight of happy couples with children gave her and which made her shun other women and their company, the fear that her husband was unfaithful (which fear was probably justified), and the lack of any fixed or definite purpose, the lack of a great pride or self-sufficiency, brought on symptoms that necessitated her removal to a sanitarium.

This of course pricked the conscience of her husband. He visited her frequently, vowed a complete change, promised to bring his business to the point where he would be able to come home at six, etc., etc. Gradually she improved and finally made a partial recovery.

Whether or not the husband kept his promises I cannot say. On the chances he did. Most confirmed gamblers, however, remain gamblers. The lure of excitement is more potent to such men than a wife whose charm has gone, through familiarity, through time itself, through the inconstancy of passion and love. The gambler usually knows no duty; he is kind and generous but only to please himself. He is easily bored and his sympathies rarely stand the disagreeable long; he knows only one *constant* attraction,— Chance.

The other woman suffered in much the same way except that she was fortunate enough finally to be deserted by her husband. This ended her doubts and fears, broke her down for a short while, and then she went back to industry. In this I have no doubt she found only an incomplete satisfaction for her yearnings and desires, but she had something to take up her time, and built up contacts with others in a way that was impossible in her lonely home.

Case IX. The will to power through weakness; a case of hysteria in the home.

This case is classic in the outspoken value of the symptoms to the woman. It is not of course typical, except as the extreme is typical, and that is what is usually meant. Roosevelt, we say, was a typical American, meaning that he represented in extreme development a certain type of man. So this case shows very clearly what is not so clear at first in many cases of conflict between man and wife.

The woman in question was twenty-seven, of French-Canadian origin, but thoroughly American in appearance and speech. She was of a middle-class rural family and had married a farmer who finally had given up his farm and was a mechanic in a small city.

The young woman had always been irritable, egoistic, and sensitive. As a girl if anything happened to "shock her nerves", *i.e.* to displease her, she fainted, vomited, or went into "hysterics." As a result her family treated her with great caution and probably were well pleased when she married off their hands and left the home.

Married life soon provided her with sufficient to displease her. Her husband drank but not sufficiently to be classed as a heavy drinker. He was a quiet, rather taciturn man, utterly averse to the pleasures for which his wife longed. She wanted to go to dances, to take in the theaters, to live in more expensive rooms, and especially she became greatly attached to a group of people of a sporty type whom her husband tersely called "tin-horn bluffs" and whom he refused to visit.

They quarreled vigorously and the quarrels always ended one way, — she became sick in one way or other. This usually brought her husband around to her way of thinking, at least for a time, and much against his will he would go with her to her friends.

Finally, however, she set her heart on living with these people, and he set his will firmly against hers. She then developed such an alarming set of symptoms that after a while the physician who asked my opinion had made up his mind that she had a brain tumor. She was paralyzed, speechless, did not eat and seemed desperately ill.

The diagnosis of hysteria was established by the absence of any evidence of organic disease and by the history of the case. The relief of symptoms was brought about by means which I need not detail here, but which essentially consisted in proving to the patient that no true paralysis existed and in tricking her into movement and speech.

When she was well enough to be up and about and to talk freely, she and her husband were both informed that the symptoms arose because her will was thwarted, and *that* part of their function was to bring the man to his knees. He agreed to this, but she took offense and refused to come any more to see me, — a not unnatural reaction.

The outlook in such a case is that the couple will live like cats and dogs. Such a temperament as this woman's is inborn. She is essentially, in the complete meaning of the word, unreasonable. Her nature demands a sympathetic attention and consideration that her character does not warrant. Throughout life she demands to receive but has no desire to give. Nor is she powerful enough to take, so there arise emotional crises with marked disturbance in bodily energy, and especially symptoms that frighten the onlooker, such as paralyses, blindness, deafness, fainting spells, etc. Whatever is the source of these symptoms, they are frequently used to gain some end or purpose through the sympathy and discomfort of others.

Not all hysteria, either in men or women, is united with such a character as this woman's. Sufficient stress and strain may bring about hysterical symptoms in a relatively normal person and short hysterical reactions are common in the normal woman. The height of cynicism may be found in the discovery that war causes hysteria in some men in much the same way that matrimony causes hysteria in some women. A humorous review of a paper on the domestic neuroses was entitled "Kitchen Shell Shock." But severe hysteria, when it arises in the housewife, springs mainly from her disposition and not from the kitchen.

Case X. The unfaithful husband.

Monogamous marriage is based upon the assumption that loyalty to a single male is moral and possible. It is probable that in no age has this agreement been loyally carried out by the husbands; it is probable that in our own time the single standard of morals has first been strongly emphasized. With the rise of women into equality one of the important demands they have made is that men remain as loyal as themselves. Therefore the reaction to unchastity or unfaithfulness on the part of the man is apt to be more severe than in the past, on the theory that where more is demanded failure in performance is felt the keener.

The housewife, Mrs. F. C., aged thirty-five, is a prepossessing woman, the mother of two children, and has been married for nine years. Her health has always been fairly good, though in the last four years she has been somewhat irritable. She attributed this to struggle to make both ends meet, her husband being a workman with wages just over the border line of sufficiency. They quarreled "no more than other couples do", were as much in love "as other couples are", to use her phrases. She was above her class in education, read what are usually called advanced books, was "strong for suffrage", etc. However she was a good housekeeper, devoted to her children and faithful to her husband. Their sexual relations were normal and up till six months before I saw her she thought herself a well-mated, rather fortunate woman.

Out of a clear sky came proof of long-continued unfaithfulness on the part of her "domestic" husband: a chance bill for women's clothes fluttered out of his pocket and under the bed, so that next morning she found it; an unbelieving moment and then a visit to the address on the bill, and proof plenty that he had been disloyal, not only to her but to the children, who had been obliged to scrimp along while he helped maintain another woman. Humiliated beyond measure by her disaster, unable to endure her past memories of happiness and faith, with an unstable world rocking before her, through the revelation that a quiet, contented, loving man could be completely false, she found no adequate reason for living and became a helpless prey to her troubled mind. "A temporary unfaithfulness, a yielding to sudden temptation" she could understand, but a determined plan of duplicity shattered her whole scheme of values. A very severe psychoneurosis followed, and her children and she were taken over by her parents and cared for.

Sleeplessness was so prominent in her case and so evidently the central physical symptom that its control was difficult and required a regular campaign for success. With sleep restored and the resumption of eating, the most of her acute symptoms were passed, though a profound depression remained.

Her husband, thoroughly abashed and ashamed, made furtive attempts at reconciliation. These were absolutely rejected, and from her attitude it was obvious that no reconciliation was possible. "Had he not been found out," said the wife, "he would still be living with her. I can never trust him again; I would die before I lived with him."

Little by little her pride recovered, for in such cases the deepest wound is to the ego, the self-valuation. The deepest effort of life is to increase that valuation by increasing its power and its respect by others; the keenest hurt comes with the lowering of the valuation of one's own personality. A woman gives herself to a man, without lowering a self-feeling if he is tender and faithful; if he holds her cheap, as by flagrant disloyalty, then her surrender is her most painful of memories.

With the recovery of pride came the restoration of her interest in her children, and her purposes reshaped themselves into definite plans. Part of the process in readjustment in any disordered life is to centralize the dispersed purposes, to redirect the life energies. She agreed that she would accept aid from the husband, as his duty, but only for the children. For herself, as soon as the children were a year or so older, she would go back to industry and become self-supporting. Her plans made, her recovery proceeded to a firm basis, and I have no doubt as to its permanence. Nevertheless, life has changed its complexion for her, and there will be many moments of agony. These are inevitable and part of the recovery process.

I shall not attempt to settle the larger problem of whether she should have forgiven her husband and returned to him. Granting that his repentance was genuine, granting that no further lapse would occur, she would never be able to forget that when he deceived her he had *acted* the part of a devoted husband. She would never be able fully to trust him, and this would spoil their married happiness entirely. "For the children's sake," cry some readers; well, that is the only strong argument for return. But on the whole it seems to me that an honest separation, an honest revolt of a proud woman is better than a dishonest reunion, or a "patient Griselda" acceptance of gross wrong.

Case XI. The unfaithful wife.

In such cases as the preceding and the one now to be detailed, the difficulties of the physician are multiplied by his entrance into ethics. Ordinarily medicine has nothing to do with morals; to the doctor saint and sinner are alike, and the only immorality is not to follow orders. To do one's duty as a doctor, with one's sole aim the physical health of the patient, may mean to advise what runs counter to the present-day code of morals.

This is the true "Doctor's Dilemma." In such cases discretion is the safest reaction, and discretion bids the physician say, "Call in some one else on that matter; I am only a doctor."

A true neurologist must regard himself as something more than a physician. He needs be a good preacher, an astute man of the world, as well as something of a lawyer. The patient expects counsel of an intimate kind, expects aid in the most difficult situations, viz., the conflicts of health and ethics.

Mrs. A. R., thirty-one years of age and very attractive, has been married since the age of eighteen. She has two children, and her husband, ten years her senior, is a man of whose character she says, "Every one thinks he is perfect." A little overstaid and overdignified, inclined to be pompous and didactic, he is kind-hearted and loyal, and successful in a small business. He is an immigrant Swiss and she is American born, of Swiss parentage.

Always romantic, Mrs. A. R. became greatly dissatisfied with her home life. At times the whole scheme of things, matrimony, settled life, got on her nerves so that she wanted to scream. She was bored, and it seemed to her that soon she would be old without ever having really lived. "I married before I had any fun, and I have n't had any fun since I married except" — Except for the incident that broke down her health by swinging her into mental channels that made her long for the quiet domesticity against which she had so rebelled. Her daydreaming was erotic, but romantically so, not realistic.

There are in the community adventurers of both sexes whose main interest in life is the conquest of some woman or man. The male sex adventurers are of two main groups, a crude group whose object is frank possession and a group best called sex-connoisseurs, who seek victims among the married or the hitherto virtuous; who plan a campaign leisurely and to whom possession must be preceded by difficulties. Frequently these gentry have been crude, but as satiation comes on a new excitement is sought in the invasion of other men's homes. Undoubtedly they have a philosophy of life that justifies them.

Since this is not a novel we may omit the method by which one of these men found his way to the secret desires of our patient, and how he proceeded to develop her dissatisfaction into momentary physical disloyalty. She came out of her dereliction dazed; could it be she who had done this, who had descended into the vilest degradation? She broke off all relations with the man, probably much to his surprise and disgust, and plunged into a self-accusatory internal debate that brought about a profound neurasthenia.

Naturally she did not of her own accord speak of her unfaithfulness, — largely because no one knew of it. Her husband did not in the least suspect her; he thought she needed a rest, a change, little realizing how "change" had broken her down. (For after all, the most of infidelity is based on a sort of curiosity, a seeking of a new stimulus, rather than true passion.) The truth was forced out of her when it was evident to me that something was obsessing her.

When she had confessed her difficulty the question arose as to her husband. She was no longer dissatisfied, no longer eager for romance; but could she live with him if she had been unfaithful? Ought she not to tell him; and yet she feared to do this, feared the result to him, for she felt sure he would forgive her. In reality the conflict in her mind arose first from self-depreciation and second from indecision as to confession.

As to the self-accusation, I told her that though she had been very foolish she had punished herself severely enough; that her reaction was that of an *essentially moral* person; that an essentially immoral woman would have continued in her career, and at least would not have been so remorseful. As to confessing, I told her that I believed that if she came to peace without such a confession wisdom would dictate not to make it, and that perhaps a little romanticism was still present in the quixotic idea of confession. Discretion is sometimes the better part of veracity, and I felt sure that she would not find it difficult to forget her pain.

It may be questioned whether such advice was ethical. I am sure no two professors of ethics could agree on the matter, and where they would disagree I chose the policy of expediency. Moreover, I felt certain that Mrs. R.'s remorse did not need the purge of confession to her husband, that she was not of that deeply fixed nature which requires heroic measures. Her confession to me was sufficient, and since it was apparent that she would not repeat her folly it was not necessary to go to extremes.

The last two cases make pertinent some further remarks on sex. It has previously been stated that the sex field is the one in which arise many of the difficulties which breed the psychoneuroses. It would not be the place here to give details of cases, though every neurologist of experience is well aware of the neuroses that arise in marriage, among both men and women. Some day society will reach the plane where matters relating to the great function by which the world is perpetuated can be discussed with the freedom allowed to the discussion of the details of nutrition.

No one seriously doubts that women are breaking away from traditional ideas in these matters. There was a time (the Victorian Age) in the United States and England when prudery ruled supreme in the manners and dress of women. That this has largely disappeared is a good thing, but whether there is a tendency to another extreme is a matter where division of opinion will occur. A transition from long skirts to dress that will permit complete freedom of movement and resembling in a feminine way the garments of men would be unqualifiedly good. It would remove undue emphasis of sex and accentuate the essential human-ness of woman. But a transition from long skirts to short tight ones, impeding movement, is the transition from prudery to pruriency and is by no means a clear gain. Plenty of scope for art and beauty might be found in a costume of which pantalettes of some kind are the basis. I doubt if women will ever be regarded quite as human beings so long as they paint, wear fantastic coiffures, hobble along on foolish heels, and are clad in overtight short skirts.

Similarly with the literature of the period. The so-called sex story, the sex problem, obsesses the writers. Nor are these frank, free discussions of the essential difficulties in the relation between man and woman. Usually the stories deal with the difficulties of the idle rich woman without children, or concern themselves with trivial triangles. In the type of interminable continued stories that every newspaper now carries, the woman's difficulties range around the most absurd petty jealousies, and she never seems to cook or sew or have any responsibility, and they always end so "sweetly." On the stage the epidemic of girl and music shows has quite displaced the drama. Here sex is exploited to the point of the risque and sometimes beyond it.

Sex is overemphasized by our civilization on its distracting side, its spicy and condimental values, and underemphasized so far as its realities go. The aim seems to be to titillate sex feeling constantly, and a precocious acquaintance with this form of stimulation is the lot of most city children. Such things would have no serious results to the housewife if they did not arouse expectations that marriage does not fulfill at all. This is the great harm of prurient clothes, literature, art, and stage, — it unfits people for sex reality.

In how far the delayed marriages of men and women are good or bad it is almost impossible to decide. That unchastity increases with delay is a certainty, that fewer children are born is without doubt. Whether the fixation of habit makes it harder for the wife to settle down to the household, and the man less domestic, cannot be answered with yes or no. There seems to be no greater wisdom of choice shown in mature than in early marriages, though this would be best answered by an analysis of divorce records.

That contraceptive measures have come to stay; that they are increasing in use, the declining birth rate absolutely evidences. I take no stock in the belief that education reduces fertility through some biological effect; where it reduces fertility it does so through a knowledge of cause, effect, and prevention. Some day it will come to pass that contraceptive measures will be legal, in view of the fact that our jurists and law makers are showing a decline in the size of their own families. When that time comes the discussion of means of this kind consistent with nervous health will be frank, and some part of the neurasthenia of our modern times will disappear. The vaster racial problems that will arise are not material for discussion in this book.

Though not perhaps completely relevant to the nervousness of the housewife, it is not without some point to touch on the "neurosis of the engaged." The freedom of the engaged couple is part of the emancipation of youth in our time. Frankly, a love-making ensues that stops just short of the ultimate relationship, an excitement and a tension are aroused and perpetuated through the frequent and protracted meetings. Sweet as this period of life is, in many cases it brings about a mild exhaustion, and in other cases, relatively few, a severe neurosis. On the whole the engagement period of the average American couple is not a good preparation for matrimony. How to bring about restraint without interfering with normal love-making is not an easy decision to make. But it would be possible to introduce into the teaching of hygiene the necessity of moderation in the engaged period; it would be especially of service to those whose engagement must be prolonged to be advised concerning the matter. Here is a place for the parents, the family friend, or the family physician.

Men and women as they enter matrimony are only occasionally equipped with real knowledge as to the physiology and psychology of the sex life. That a great deal of domestic dissatisfaction and unhappiness could be obviated if wisdom and experience instructed the husband and wife in the matter I have not the slightest doubt. The first rift in the domestic lute often dates from difficulties in the intimate life of the pair, difficulties that need not exist if there were knowledge. That reason and love may coexist, that the beauty of life is not dependent on a sentimentalized ignorance are cardinal in my code of beliefs. He who believes that sentiment disappears with enlightenment is the true cynic, the true pessimist. He who believes that intelligence and knowledge should guide instinct and that happiness is thus more certain is better than an optimist; he is a rationalist, a realist.

CHAPTER XII

Treatment of the Individual Cases

It is obvious that what is largely a problem of the times cannot be wholly considered as an individual problem. Yet individual cases do yield to treatment (to use the slang of medicine) or at least a large proportion do. The minor cases in point of symptoms are very frequently the most stubborn, since neither the patient nor the family are willing to concede that to alter the life situation is as important as the taking of medicine.

Most housewives are nervous, both in their own eyes and in those of their husbands, yet rightly they are not regarded as sick. They are uncomfortable, even unhappy, and the way out seems impossible to find. I believe that even with things as they are, adjustments are possible that can help the average woman. It is conceded that where the life situation involves an unalterable factor, relief or help may be unobtainable.

It is necessary first of all to rule out physical disease. To do this means a thorough physical study. By doing this a considerable number of women will be immensely helped. Flat feet, varicose veins, injuries to the organs of generation, eye strain, relaxed gastro-intestinal tract, and the major diseases, — these must be remembered as factors that may determine nervousness.

With this question settled, let us assume that there is no such difficulty or it has been remedied, and we have next to consider the life situation of the patient. Here we enter into a difficult place, where knowledge of life and understanding of men and women, as well as tact, are the essentials.

It is necessary to remedy whatever bad hygienic habits exist. A rich woman may have settled down to a deënergizing life, with too much time in bed, too many matinées, too many late nights, too many bonbons, etc. Aside from the psychical injuries that such a life produces, it is bad for "the nerves" in its effects upon digestion, bodily tone, and the sources of mood. On some simple detail of life, some unfortunate habit, the whole structure of misery may rest.

I always keep in mind an incident of some years ago when I lived in a small town in Massachusetts. For some reason our furnace threw coal gas into the house in such a way as nearly to poison us. The landlord sent several plumbers down, and one after the other suggested drastic remedies, — a new chimney, a new furnace, etc. Finally the landlord and I investigated for ourselves. At the bottom of the chimney we found an inconspicuous loose brick which allowed air to enter the chimney beneath the entrance of the pipe from the stove. We got ten cents' worth of lime and fastened the brick in firmly. A complete cure, where the specialists had failed.

So there often exists some drain on the energy and strength of the woman which may be simple and easily changed, and yet is critical in its significance and importance.

An overdomestic woman may stick too closely to the house; an underdomestic one may go too often to movies and suffer the fatigue of mind and body that comes from over-indulgence in this most popular indoor sport. Carelessness about the eating and the care of the bowel functions may have started a vicious chain of things leading through irritability and fatigue into neurasthenia. We say human beings are all the same, but the range of individual susceptibility to trouble is such that a difficulty not important to most people will raise havoc with others who are in most ways perfectly normal.

Look then for the bad hygiene! Look for the evils of the sedentary life Look for the root of the trouble in lack of exercise, poor habits of eating, insufficient air, disturbed sleep! Search for physical difficulties before inquiring into the psychical life.

If poverty exists, then one may inquire into the amount of work done, the character of the home, the opportunities for recreation and recuperation. All or any of the factors I have mentioned in previous chapters may be critical, and the moil and turmoil of a crowded tenement home may be responsible. That such conditions do not break all women down does not prove that they do not break *some* women down, women with finer sensibilities, or lesser endurance (which often go together). The most depressing problems are met among the poor, the cases where one can see no way out because the social machinery is inadequate to care for its victims.

What is one to do when one meets a poor woman with three or four or more children, living in a crowded way, overworked, racked in her nerves by her fears, worries, and the disagreeable in her life, drudging from morning till night, yearning for better things, despairing of getting them, tormented by desires and ambitions that must be thwarted? "What right has a poor woman anyway to desires above her station, and why does not she resign herself to her lot?" ask the comfortable. Unfortunately philosophy and resignation are difficult even for philosophers and saints, and much more so for the aspiring woman. And our American civilization preaches "Strive, Strive!" too constantly for much philosophy and resignation of an effective kind to be found.

One must give tonics, prescribe rest, try to get social agencies interested, obtain vacations and convalescent care, etc. Can one purge a woman of futile longings and strivings, rid her of natural fears and even of absurd fears? It can be done to a limited degree, if the patient has intelligence and if one gives liberally of one's time and sympathy. But unfortunately the consulting room for the poor is in the crowded clinic, the thronged dispensary, and how is the overworked physician to give the time and energy necessary?

For the time required is the least requirement. To deal adequately with the neurasthenic is to have unending sympathy and patience and an energy that is limitless. Without such energy or endurance the physician either slumps to a prescriber of tonics and sedatives, a dispenser of such stale advice as "Don't worry" and "You need a rest", or else himself gives out.

In dealing with the cases in the better-to-do and the rich, one has more weapons in the armamentarium. The worry is more futile here, more ridiculous, and one can attack it vigorously. Usually it is not overwork in these cases; it is monotony, boredom, discontent with something or other, a vicious circle of depressing thoughts and emotions, some difficulty in the sex life, some reaction against the husband, a rebellion of a weak, futile kind against life, maladjustment of a temperament to a situation.

Some difficulties, even when ascertained and clearly understood, are insurmountable. "The truth shall make ye free" is true only in the very largest sense. Some temperaments are inborn, and are as unchangeable as the nose on one's face. In such cases the ordinary physical therapeutics help the acute symptoms that flare up now and then, and that is as much as one may expect.

But it is certain that in the majority of cases more than this may be accomplished. It is often a great surprise and relief to a woman to realize that her overconscientiousness, her fussiness, her rebellion, and discontent, her reaction to something or other is back of her symptoms. She has feared disease of the brain, tumor, insanity, or has blamed her trouble on some other definite physical basis.

If one deals with intelligence, explanation helps a great deal. The intelligent usually want to be convinced; they do not ask for miracles, they seek counsel as well as treatment.

It is my firm belief that the function of intelligence is to control instinct and emotion, and that temperament, if inborn, is not unchangeable, even at maturity. Once you convince a person that his or her symptoms are due to fear, worry, doubt, and rebellion you enlist the personal efforts to change.

A new philosophy of life must be presented.

Less fussiness, less fear, more endurance, less reaction to the trifles of their life are necessary. The aimless drifter must be given a central purpose or taught to seek one; the dissatisfied and impatient must be asked, "Why should life give you all you want?" "What cannot be remedied must be endured!" What a wealth of wisdom in the proverb! One seeks to establish an ideal of fortitude, of patience, of fidelity to duty, — old-fashioned words, but serenity of spirit is their meaning. Suddenly to come face to face with one's self, to strip away the self-imposed disguise, to see clearly that jealousy, impatience, luxurious, and never satisfied tastes, a selfish and restless spirit, are back of ennui and fatigue, pains and aches of body and mind, is to step into a true self-understanding.

If a situation demands action, even drastic action, "surgical" action, then that action must be forthcoming, even though it hurts. To end doubt, perplexity, to cease being buffeted between hither and yon, is to end an intolerable life situation. I have in mind certain domestic situations, such as the effort to keep up in appearance and activity with those of more means and ability.

Sexual difficulties, so important and so common, demand the coöperation of the husband for remedy. He should be seen (for usually the wife consults the physician alone) and the situation gone over with him. Men are usually willing to help, willing to seek a way out. A neurasthenic wife is a sore trial to the patience and endurance of her husband and he is anxious enough to help cure her.

Where there is conflict of other kinds the situation is complicated by the intricacy of the factors. Financial difficulties especially wear down the patience and endurance of the partners, and the physician cannot prescribe a golden cure. In prosperous times there is less neurasthenia than in the unprosperous, just as there is less suicide.

Sometimes it is just one thing, one difficulty, over which the conflict rages. I have in mind two such cases, where one habit of the husband deënergized his wife by outraging her pride and love. When he was induced to yield on this point the wife came back to herself, — a highly strung, very efficient self.

In fact, the basis of treatment is the painstaking study of the individual woman and then the painstaking *adjustment* of that individual woman. It may mean the adjustment of the whole life situation to that housewife, or conversely the adjustment of the housewife to the life situation.

In many marital difficulties that one sees, not so much in practice as in contact with normal married couples, the trouble reminds one of the orang-outang in Kipling's story who had "too much Ego in his Cosmos." Marriage, to be successful, is based on a graceful recession of the ego in the cosmos of each of the partners. The prime difficulty is this; people do not like to recede the ego. And the worst offenders are the ones who are determined to stand up for the right, which usually is a disguised way of naming their desire.

One might speak of a thousand and one things that every man and every woman knows. One might speak of the death of love and the growth of irritation, the disappearance of sympathy, — these are the hopeless situations. But far more common and important, though less tragic, is the disappearance of the little attentions, the little lovemaking, the disappearance of good manners. Men are not the only or the worst offenders in this; the nervous housewife is very apt to be the scold and the nag. Perhaps the neurasthenia of the husband arises from his revolt against the incessant demands of his wife, but that 's another story.

At any rate, there is what seems to be a cardinal point of difference between men and women, perhaps arising from some essential difference in make-up, perhaps in part due to difference in training. An essential need of the average American-trained woman is sympathy, constantly expressed, constantly manifested. The average man tends to become matter-of-fact, the average woman finds in matter-of-factness the death of love. She acts as if she believed that the little acts of love and sympathy are the more important as manifesting the real state of feeling, that the major duties were of less importance.

On this point most men and women never seem to agree. The man gets impatient over the constant demand for his attention. He thinks it unreasonable and childish. Intent upon his own struggle he is apt to think her affairs are minor matters. He thinks his wife makes mountains out of molehills and lacks a sense of proportion. He forgets that the devotion of the husband is the woman's anchor to windward, her grip on safety, — that his success and struggle are hers only in so far as he and she are intimate and lover-like. And women, even those who trust their husbands absolutely so far as physical loyalty goes, jealously watch them for the appearance of boredom, or lack of interest, for the falling off of the lover's spirit and feeling.

After marriage the rivalry of men expresses itself in business more than in love. Even where a woman does not fear another woman as a rival she fears the rivalry of business, — and with reason. So she craves attention, sympathy, as well as the dull love of everyday life. She ought to have it; it is her recompense for her lot, for her married life, her smaller interests. Now and then some great man intent upon a great work has some excuse for absorption in that work; for the great majority of men there is no such excuse. Their own affairs are also minor and are no more important than those of their wives. Fair play demands that the women they have immured in a home have a prior claim to their company, in at least the majority of the leisure hours. If in the time to come the home alters and a woman who continues to work marries a man who works, and they meet only at night, then it will be ethical for each to go his or her way. Marriage at present must mean the giving up of freedom for the man as well as for the woman, in the interests of justice and the race.

In medicine we prescribe bitter tonics which have the property of increasing appetite and vigor. For the husband of every woman there is this bit of advice; sympathy and attention constitute a sweet tonic, which if judiciously administered is of incomparable power and efficiency.

CHAPTER XIII

The Future of Woman, the Home, and Marriage

No true sportsman ever prophesies. For the odds are overwhelmingly in favor of the prophet. If he is right, he can brag the rest of his days of his seer-like vision. If he is wrong, no one takes the trouble to reproach or mock him.

Therefore I do not claim to be a prophet in discussing the future of woman, the home, and marriage. At any time just one invention may come along that will totally alter the face of things. Moreover we are now in the midst of great changes in industry, in social relations, in the largest matters of national and international nature. Men and women alike are involved in these changes, but it is impossible to judge the outcome. For history records many abortive reformations, many reactionary centuries and eras as well as successful reformations and progressive ages.

Whether or not it fits woman to be a housewife of the traditional kind, feminism is certain to develop further. Women will enter into more diverse occupations than ever before, they will enter politics, they will find their way to direct power and action. More and more those who work will be specialized and individualized — the woman executive, the writer, the artist, the doctor, lawyer, architect, chemist, and sociologist — will resist the dictum "Woman's place is the Home." The woman of this group will either be forced into celibacy, or in ever-increasing numbers she will insist on some sort of arrangement whereby she can carry on her work. She will perhaps refuse to bear children and transform domesticity into an apartment hotel life, in which she and her husband eat breakfast and dinner together and spend the rest of the waking time separately, as two men might.

Such a development, while perhaps satisfying the ideas of progress of the feminist, will be bad eugenically. There will be a removal from the race of the value of these women, the intellectual members of their sex.

Whether the work this group of women do will equal the value of the children they might have had no one can say.

But after all, the number of women who will enter the professions and remain in them on the conditions above stated will be relatively small. The main function of women will always be childbearing. If ever there comes a time when the drift will be away from this function, then a counter-movement will start up to sway women back into this sphere of their functions. Moreover, the bulk of women entering industry will enter it in the humbler occupations and they will in the main be willing enough to marry and bear children, even in the limited way. Yet since they enter marriage with a wider experience than ever before, the conditions of marriage and the home must change, even though gradually.

So on the whole we may look to an increasing individuality of woman, an increasing feeling of worth and dignity as an individual, an increasing reluctance to take up life as the traditional housewife. Rebellion against the monotony and the seclusive character of the home will increase rather than diminish, and it must be faced without prejudice and without any reliance on any authority, either of church or state, that will force women back to "womanly" ways of thinking, feeling or doing.

Sooner or later we shall have to accept legally what we now recognize as fact, — the restriction of childbearing. Whether we regard it as good or bad, the modern woman will not bear and nurse a large family. And the modern man, though he has his little joke about the modern family, is one with his wife in this matter. With husband and wife agreed there seems little to do but accept the situation.

That this condition of affairs is leaving the peopling of the world to the backward, the ignorant, and the careless is at present accepted by most authors. One has only to read the serious articles on this subject in the journals devoted to racial biology to realize how deeply important the matter is. Yet there may be some undue alarm felt, for contraceptive measures are becoming so prevalent in Europe, America, and Asia that all races will soon be on the same footing, and moreover all classes in society except the feeble-minded are learning the procedures. The prolificness of the feeble-minded is indeed a menace, and society may find itself compelled to lower their fertility artificially.

What will probably happen is that the one, two, or three-child family will be born before the mother's thirty-fifth year, and she will then or before forty become free from the severest burdens of the housewife. What will she do with her time; what will the better-to-do woman do? Will she gradually give her energies to the community, or will she while away her time in the spurious culture that occupies so many club women to-day?

It is safe to say that women will enter far more largely than ever before into movements for the betterment of the race. Though their way of life may breed neurasthenia for some, it will have this great advantage,— the mother feeling will sweep into society, will enter politics, and social discussions. That we need that feeling no one will deny who has ever tried to enlist social energies for race betterment and failed while politicians stepped in for all the funds necessary even for some anti-social activities. We have too much legalism in our social structure and not near enough of the humanism that the socially minded mother can bring.

Is the increasing incidence of divorce a revolt against domesticity? To some extent yes, but where women obtain the divorce it is mainly a refusal to tolerate unfaithfulness, desertion, incompatibility of temperament. It does not mean that the family is threatened by divorce, — rather that the family is threatened by the conditions for which divorce is nowadays obtained and which were formerly not reasons for divorce. In many countries adultery on the part of the man, cruel and abusive treatment, chronic intoxication, and desertion were not grounds for divorce. These to-day are the grounds for divorce, and in the opinion of the writer they should invalidate a marriage. I would go even further and say that wherever there was concealed insanity or venereal disease the marriage should be annulled, as it is in some States.

Divorce will not then diminish, despite the campaign against it, until the conditions for which it is sought are removed. Until that time comes, to bind two people together who are manifestly unhappy simply encourages unfaithfulness and cruelty, and is itself a cruelty.

Whether we can devise a system where woman's individuality and humanness can have scope and yet find her willing to accept the rôles of mother and homekeeper, is a serious question. It seems to me certain that woman will continue to demand her freedom, regardless of her status as wife and mother. She will continue to receive more and more general and special education, and she will continue to find the rôle of the traditional housewife more uncongenial. Out of that maladaptation and the discontent and rebellion will arise her neurosis.

In other words what we must seek to do — those of us who are not bound by tradition alone but who seek to modify institutions to human beings rather than the reverse — is to find out what changes in the home and matrimonial conditions are necessary for the woman of to-day and to-morrow.

That there has been a huge migration to the cities in the last century is one of its outstanding peculiarities. This urban movement has meant the greater concentration of humans in a given area, and it is therefore directly responsible for the apartment house. That is to say, there has been a trend away from individual homes, completely segregated and individualized, to houses where at least part of the housework was eliminated, in a sense was coöperative. This coöperation is increasing; more and more houses have janitors, more and more houses furnish heat. In the highest class of apartment house the trend is toward permanent hotel life, with the exception that individual housekeeping is possible.

Because of the limited space and the desire of the modern well-to-do woman to escape as much as possible from housekeeping, because of the smaller families (which idea has been fostered by landlords), the number of rooms and the size of the rooms have grown less. The kitchenette apartment is a new departure for those who can afford more room, for it is well known that the poor in the slums have long since lived in one or two rooms serving all purposes. The huge modern apartment house, the huge modern tenement house, are part first of the urban movement and second of that movement away from housekeeping which has been sketched in the Introduction.

The home has been praised as the nucleus of society, its center, its heart. Its virtues have been so unanimously extolled that one need but recite them. It is the embodiment of family, the soul of mother, father, and children. It is the place where morality and modesty are taught. In it arise the basic virtues of love of parents, love of children, love of brothers and sisters; sympathy is thus engendered; loyalty has here its source. The privacy of the home is a refuge from excitement and struggle and gives rest and peace to the weary battler with the world. It is a sanctuary where safety is to be sought, and this finds expression in the English proverb, "Every Englishman's home is his castle." It is a reward, a purpose in that men and women dream of their own home and are thrilled by the thought. Throughout its quiet runs the scarlet thread of its sex life. Home is where love is legitimate and encouraged.

Yet the home has great faults; it is no more a divine institution than anything else human is. Without at all detracting from its great, its indispensable virtues, let us, as realists, study its defects.

On the physical-economic side is the inefficiency and waste inseparable from individual housekeeping. Labor-saving machinery and devices are often too expensive for the individual home, and so small stoves do the cooking and the heating, each individual housewife or her helper washes by hand the dishes of each little group. Shopping is a matter for each woman, and necessitates numberless small shops; perhaps the biggest waste of time and energy lies here. The cooking is done according to the intelligence and knowledge of nutrition of each housewife, and housewives, like the rest of the world, range in intelligence from feeble-mindedness to genius, with a goodly number of the uninformed, unintelligent, and careless. Poets and novelists and the stage extol home cooking, but the doctors and dietitians know there are as many kinds of home cooking as there are kinds of homekeepers. The laboratory and not the home has been the birthplace of the science of nutrition, and we have still many traditions regarding the merits of home cooking and feeding to break from.

Take as one minor example the gorging

encouraged on Sunday and certain holidays. The housewife feels it her duty to slave in a kitchen all Sunday morning that an over-big meal may be eaten in half an hour by her family. She encourages gluttony by feeling that her standing as cook is directly proportional to the heartiness of her meal. Thanksgiving, Christmas, — the good cheer of gluttony is sentimentalized and hallowed into poetry and music. The table that groans under its good cheer has its sequence in the diners who groan without cheer.

While we might further dilate on the physical deficiencies and inefficiencies of the segregated home, there is a disadvantage of vaster importance. After all, institutionalized cooking is rarely satisfactory, because it lacks the spirit of good home cooking, the desire to meet individual taste without profit. It lacks the ideal of service.

There are bad effects from the segregation and the privacy of the home, even of the good kind. For there are very many bad homes; those in which drunkenness, immorality, quarreling, selfishness, improvidence, brutality, and crime are taught by example. After all, we like to speak too much in generalities — the Home, Woman, Man, Labor, Capital, Mankind — forgetting there is no such thing as "the Home." There are homes of all kinds with every conceivable ideal of life and training and having only one thing in common, — that they are segregated social units, based usually on the family relationship. Montaigne very truly said approximately this: "He who generalizes says 'Hello' to a crowd; he who *knows* shakes hands with individuals."

In the first place the home (to show my inconsistency in regard to generalizing) is the place where prejudice is born, nourished, and grown to its fullest proportions. The child born and reared in a home is exposed to the contagion of whatever silliness and prejudice actuate the lives and dominate the thought and feeling of its parents. And the quirks and twists to which it is exposed affect its life either positively or negatively, for it either accepts their prejudices or develops counter-prejudices against them. To cite a familiar case; it is traditional that some of the children brought up overstrictly, overcarefully, throw off as soon as possible and as completely as possible conventional morals and manners. Such persons have simply overreacted to their training, revolted against the prejudice of their teaching by building counter-prejudices.

Further, the home fosters an anti-social feeling, or perhaps it would be kinder to say a non-social feeling. Your home-loving person comes in the course of time to that state of mind where little else is of importance; the home becomes the only place where his sympathies and his altruistic purposes find any real outlet. The capitalist of the stage (and of real life too) is one so devoted to his home and family that he decorates one and the other with the trophies of other homes. There is none so devoted to his home as the peasant, and there is no one so individualistic, so intent in his own prosperity. The home encourages an intense altruism, but usually a narrow one. The feeling of warmth and comfort of the hearth fire when a blizzard rages outside too often makes us forget the poor fellows in the blizzard.

Thus the home is the backbone of conservatism, which is good, but it becomes also the basis of reactionary feeling. It is the people that break away from home and home ties who do the great things.

When the home is quiet and harmonious it is the place where great virtues are developed. But when it is noisy and disharmonious, then its very seclusiveness, its segregation, lends to the quarrels the bitterness of civil war. The intensity of feeling aroused is proportional to the intimacy of the home and not to the importance of the thing quarreled about. Good manners and that sign and symbol of largeness of spirit, tolerance for the opinions of others, rarely are born in the home.

It is hardly realized how much quarreling, how much of intense emotional violence goes on in many homes. Its isolation and the absence of the restraining influence of formality and courtesy bring the wills of the family members into sharp conflict. Words are used that elsewhere would bring the severest physical answer, or bring about the most complete disruption of friendly relations. Love and anger, duty and self-interest bring about intense inner conflict in the home, and the struggle between the two generations, the rising and the receding, is here at its height.

That courtesy to each other might be

taught the children, might be insisted on by the parents is my firm belief. Love and intimacy need not exclude form. Manners and morals are not exclusive of each other. If the marriage ceremony included the vow to be polite, it might leave out almost everything else. The home should be the place where tolerance, courtesy, and emotional control are taught both by precept and example.

Can the home be altered to bring in more of the social spirit and yet maintain its great virtues, its extraordinary attraction for the human heart? It 's an old story that criticism, the pointing out of defect, is easy, while good suggestions are few and difficult to convert into programs for action. In medicine diagnosis is far ahead of treatment, — so in society at large.

Any plans that have for their end a sort of social barracks, with men and women and their children living in apartments, but eating and drinking in large groups, will meet the fiercest resistance from the sentiment of our times and cannot succeed, unless it is forced on us by some breakdown of the social structure. Nevertheless a larger coöperation, at least in the cities, will come. Buildings must be built so that a deal of individual labor disappears. Just as coöperative stores are springing up, so coöperative kitchens, community kitchens organized for service would be a great benefit. Especially for the poor, without servants, where the woman is frequently forced to neglect her own rest and the children's welfare because she must cook, would such a development be of great value. Unfortunately the few community kitchens now operating have in mind only the middle-class housewife and not the housewife in most need, — the poor housewife. Here is a plan for real social service; cooking for the poor of the cities, scientific, nutritious, tasty, at cost. Much of the work of medicine would be eliminated with one stroke; much of racial degeneracy and misery would disappear in a generation.

That the home needs labor-saving devices in order that much of the disagreeable work may be eliminated is unquestioned. Inventive genius has only given a fragmentary attention to the problems of the housewife. Most of the devices in use are far beyond the means of the poor and even the lower middle class. Furthermore, though they save labor many of them do not save time. The tests by which the good household device ought to be judged are these:

First — Is it efficient?

Second — Is it labor saving?

Third — Is it time saving?

We need to break away from traditional cooking apparatus and traditional diet. The installation and use of fireless cookers, self-regulating ovens, is a first step. The discarding of most of the puddings, roasts, fancy dishes that take much time in the preparation and that keep the housewife in the kitchen would not only save the housewife but would also be of great benefit to her husband. The cult of hearty eating, which results in keeping a woman (mistress or maid) in the kitchen for three or more hours that a man may eat for twenty or thirty minutes is folly. The type of meal that either takes only a short time for preparation and devices which render the attention of the housewife unnecessary are ethical and healthy, both for the family and society. The joys of the table are not to be despised, and only the dyspeptic or the ascetic hold them in contempt; but simplicity in eating is the very heart of the joy of the table.

Elaboration and gluttony are alike in this, — they increase the housework and decrease the well-being of the diner.

How to maintain the sweetness of the family spirit of the home and yet bring into it a wider social spirit, break down its isolated individualistic character, is a problem I do not pretend to be able to solve. Ancient nations emphasized the social-national aspect of life overmuch, as for example the Spartans; the modern home overemphasizes the family aspect. We must avoid extremes by clinging to the virtues and correcting the vices of the home.

Alarmists are constantly raising the cry that marriage is declining and that society is thereby threatened at its very heart. There is the pessimist who feels that the "irreligion" of to-day is responsible; there is the one who blames feminism; and there is the type that finds in Democracy and liberalism generally the cause of the receding old-fashioned morality. Divorce, late marriage, and child-restriction are the manifestations of this decadence, and the press, the pulpit, science, and the State all have taken notice of these modern phenomena, though with widely differing attitudes.

That matrimony is changing cannot be questioned or denied. The main change is that woman is entering more and more as an equal partner whose rights the modern law recognizes as the ancient law did not. She is no longer to be classed as exemplified by the famous words of Petruchio, when he claimed his wife, the erstwhile shrew, as his property in exactly the same sense as any domestic animal, linking the wife with the horse, the cow, the ass, as the chattels of the man. The law agreed to this attitude of the man, the Church supported it; woman, strangely enough, seemed to glory in it.

With the rise of woman into the status of a human being (a revolution not yet accomplished in entirety) the property relationship weakened but lingers very strongly as a tradition that molds the lives of husband and wife. Women are still held more rigidly to their duties as wives than men to their duties as husbands, and the will of the husband still rules in the major affairs of life, even though in a thousand details the wife rules. Theoretically every man willingly acknowledges the importance of his wife as mother and homekeeper, but practically he acts as if his work were the really important activity of the family. The obedience of the wife is still asked for by most of the religious ceremonies of the times. Two great opinions are therefore still struggling in the home and in society; one that matrimony implies the dependence and essential inferiority of woman, and the other that the man and woman are equal partners in the relationship. I fully realize that the advocate of the first opinion will deny that the inferiority of woman is at all implied in their standpoint. But it is an inferior who vows obedience, it is the inferior who loses legal rights, it is the inferior who yields to another the "headship" of the home.

The struggle of these two opinions will have only one outcome, the complete victory of the modern belief that the sexes are, all in all, equal, and that therefore marriage is a contract of equals. Meanwhile the struggling opinions, with the scene of conflict in every home, in every heart, cause disorder as all struggles do. When the victory is complete, then conduct will be definite and clear-cut, then the home will be reorganized in relation to the new belief, and then new problems will arise and be met. How conduct will be changed, what the new problems will be and how they will be met, I do not pretend to know.

Meanwhile there is this to say, — that marriage should be guarded so that the grossly unfit do not marry. A thorough physical examination is as necessary for matrimony as it is for civil service, and many of the horrors every generation of doctors has witnessed could be eliminated at once and for all time.

Further, if marriage is a desirable state, and on the whole it must be preferred to a single existence, surely so long as our code of morals remains unchanged, and so long as we believe the race must be perpetuated, then the too late marriage should be discouraged. The ideal age for women to enter matrimony is from twenty-two to twenty-five; the ideal age for men is from twenty-five to twenty-eight. It is not my province to deal at length with this subject, but I may state that I believe that continence beyond these ages becomes increasingly difficult, that immorality is encouraged, that adaptability becomes lessened, and that wiser selection of mates does *not* occur. But how bring about early marriages in a time when the luxuries seem to have become necessities, and therefore the necessity of marriage is eyed more and more as an extravagance of the foolhardy? How bring about early marriage when women are earning pay almost equal to that of the men and are therefore more reluctant to enter matrimony unless at a high standard of living. The late marriage is an evil, but how it can be displaced by the early marriage under the present social scheme I do not see.

We have considered divorce before this. It is not an evil but a symptom of evil; not a disease in itself. It cannot be lessened or abolished unless we are willing to state that a man and a woman should live together as husband and wife, hating, despising, or fearing one another. We cannot countenance brutality, unfaithfulness, or temperamental mismating. It is true that divorces are often obtained for trivial reasons, but usually the partners are not adapted to one another, according to modern ways of thinking and feeling. What is commonplace in one age is cruelty in the next, and this is a matter not of argument but of expectation and feeling.

Nothing more need be said of contraceptive measures than this: they are inevitably increasing in use and soon will be part of the average marriage. Society must recognize this, and the lawmakers must legalize what they themselves practise.

Matrimony, the home, woman, these are nodal points in the network of our human lives. But they are not fixed centers, and the great weaver, Time, changes the design constantly. Through them run the threads of the great instincts, of tradition, of economic change, of the ideas, ideals, and activities of man the restless. Man will always love woman, woman will always love man; children will be born and reared, and sex conflict, maladjustment, will always be secondary to these great facts. How men and women will live together, how they will arrange for the children, will be questions that women will help the world answer as well as their mates. That the main trend of things is for better, more ethical, more just relationship, I do not doubt. The secondary, most noisy changes are perhaps evil, the main primary change is good.

Meanwhile in the hurly-burly of new things, of complex relationships, working blindly, is the nervous housewife. This book has been written that she may know herself better and thus move towards the light; that her husband may win sympathy and understanding and be bound to her in a closer, better union, and that the physician and Society may seek the direct and the remote means to helping her.

INDEX

INDEX

American Women: Images and Realities

An Arno Press Collection

[Adams, Charles F., editor]. **Correspondence between John Adams and Mercy Warren Relating to Her "History of the American Revolution," July-August, 1807.** With a new appendix of specimen pages from the **"History."** 1878.

[Arling], Emanie Sachs. **"The Terrible Siren": Victoria Woodhull, (1838-1927).** 1928.

Beard, Mary Ritter. **Woman's Work in Municipalities.** 1915.

Blanc, Madame [Marie Therese de Solms]. **The Condition of Woman in the United States.** 1895.

Bradford, Gamaliel. **Wives.** 1925.

Branagan, Thomas. **The Excellency of the Female Character Vindicated.** 1808.

Breckinridge, Sophonisba P. **Women in the Twentieth Century.** 1933.

Campbell, Helen. **Women Wage-Earners.** 1893.

Coolidge, Mary Roberts. **Why Women Are So.** 1912.

Dall, Caroline H. **The College, the Market, and the Court.** 1867.

[D'Arusmont], Frances Wright. **Life, Letters and Lectures: 1834, 1844.** 1972.

Davis, Almond H. **The Female Preacher, or Memoir of Salome Lincoln.** 1843.

Ellington, George. **The Women of New York.** 1869.

Farnham, Eliza W[oodson]. **Life in Prairie Land.** 1846.

Gage, Matilda Joslyn. **Woman, Church and State.** [1900].

Gilman, Charlotte Perkins. **The Living of Charlotte Perkins Gilman.** 1935.

Groves, Ernest R. **The American Woman.** 1944.

Hale, [Sarah J.] **Manners; or, Happy Homes and Good Society All the Year Round.** 1868.

Higginson, Thomas Wentworth. **Women and the Alphabet.** 1900.

Howe, Julia Ward, editor. **Sex and Education.** 1874.

La Follette, Suzanne. **Concerning Women.** 1926.

Leslie, Eliza. **Miss Leslie's Behaviour Book: A Guide and Manual for Ladies.** 1859.

Livermore, Mary A. **My Story of the War.** 1889.

Logan, Mrs. John A. (Mary S.) **The Part Taken By Women in American History.** 1912.

McGuire, Judith W. (A Lady of Virginia). **Diary of a Southern Refugee, During the War.** 1867.

Mann, Herman. **The Female Review: Life of Deborah Sampson.** 1866.

Meyer, Annie Nathan, editor. **Woman's Work in America.** 1891.

Myerson, Abraham. **The Nervous Housewife.** 1927.

Parsons, Elsie Clews. **The Old-Fashioned Woman.** 1913.

Porter, Sarah Harvey. **The Life and Times of Anne Royall.** 1909.

Pruette, Lorine. **Women and Leisure: A Study of Social Waste.** 1924.

Salmon, Lucy Maynard. **Domestic Service.** 1897.

Sanger, William W. **The History of Prostitution.** 1859.

Smith, Julia E. **Abby Smith and Her Cows.** 1877.

Spencer, Anna Garlin. **Woman's Share in Social Culture.** 1913.

Sprague, William Forrest. **Women and the West.** 1940.

Stanton, Elizabeth Cady. **The Woman's Bible** Parts I and II. 1895/1898.

Stewart, Mrs. Eliza Daniel. **Memories of the Crusade.** 1889.

Todd, John. **Woman's Rights.** 1867. [Dodge, Mary A.] (Gail Hamilton, pseud.) **Woman's Wrongs.** 1868.

Van Rensselaer, Mrs. John King. **The Goede Vrouw of Mana-ha-ta.** 1898.

Velazquez, Loreta Janeta. **The Woman in Battle.** 1876.

Vietor, Agnes C., editor. **A Woman's Quest: The Life of Marie E. Zakrzewska, M.D.** 1924.

Woodbury, Helen L. Sumner. **Equal Suffrage.** 1909.

Young, Ann Eliza. **Wife No. 19.** 1875.